My Pregnancy Recipes and Meal Planner

My Pregnancy Recipes and Meal Planner

Dr Rana Conway, RNutr
(Public Health)

white
LADDER

My Pregnancy Recipes and Meal Planner

This first edition published in 2014 by White Ladder Press, an imprint of
Crimson Publishing Ltd, 19-21c Charles Street, Bath BA1 1HX

© Rana Conway 2014

British Library Cataloguing in Publication Data
A catalogue record for this book is available from the British Library.

ISBN 978 1 908281 92 0

Typeset by IDS UK (DataConnections) Ltd
Printed and bound in Malta by Gutenberg Press Ltd

Contents

Contents

About the author

Rana Conway is a Registered Nutritionist and a member of the Nutrition Society. Over the past 20 years she has established herself as an expert in nutrition for pregnancy and childhood. She has carried out nutrition research at leading universities and her work with pregnant women earned her a PhD in 1997.

Rana has also lectured on a wide range of undergraduate courses and taught nutrition to medical students, midwives and trainee dieticians. She is the author of *What To Eat When You're Pregnant, What To Eat When You're Pregnant and Vegetarian, Weaning Made Easy* and *Weaning Made Easy Recipes.*

She lives in London with her husband and three children.

Acknowledgements

Many thanks to Beth Bishop, Rachael Anderson and Susi Elmer at White Ladder for all their help and enthusiasm for the book. Also to Jane Graham Maw and Jennifer Christie at Graham Maw Christie, and my husband, Olly, for his support and encouragement.

A very big thank you to everyone who tested recipes and gave invaluable feedback: Mary Arbuthnot, Victoria Axe, Katherine Brewer, Britt Burnett, Daniel Conway, Gill Conway, Joseph Conway, Madeleine Conway, Nick Conway, Penny Douglas, Jonathan Drake, Angela Farmer, Sarah Fryer, Caroline Gower, Denise Hickey, Magda Ibrahim, Rebecca Jayasinghe, Pat Lodge, Rebecca Laura, Louise Marsh, Alice Odin, Kerry Porritt and Lara Wilson.

Introduction

When you become pregnant your nutritional needs increase. Eating well will ensure you and your developing baby get all the nutrients needed for optimal growth, development and well-being. In the first section of this book, you'll find all the basics, including how your diet will affect your baby, which foods you need to avoid and what you need to eat to get all those important nutrients such as protein, iron and calcium. There's also advice about how to ensure you put on a healthy amount of weight, not too little but not too much.

The next three sections include tasty recipes to help you put all this advice into practice. The recipes are arranged by stage of pregnancy to suit your nutritional needs, but also to take into account how you're likely to be feeling. So if you're suffering from morning sickness or feeling incredibly tired in the first trimester, you'll find recipes to help. Likewise, if you want comfort food or something reasonably healthy to satisfy those cravings for sweet or sour foods, it's all there. As you settle into your pregnancy and progress to the second trimester there are plenty of low GI recipes to help you achieve a healthy weight gain, as well as prune recipes to keep constipation at bay and a few treats such as chocolate mousse, without the raw eggs of course.

Recipes for the third trimester include curries that taste fantastic, even if they don't bring on labour, healthy snacks to supply the extra calories you need at this stage and something to help if you're suffering from heartburn. There are also soups and stews to put in the freezer in preparation for the inevitably busy days ahead once your baby arrives. Scattered among the recipes you'll also find information about cravings, ginger, tuna, iron and much more to help you separate facts from old wives' tales.

The final section of the book has recipes for breastfeeding. As well as being tasty, healthy and supplying the extra calories and calcium you need at this stage, most of these are quick and easy – allowing you time to admire and bond with your new baby, and catch up on sleep when you have the chance.

Although the recipes are arranged by trimester, there's no reason you can't choose meals from other sections. If you're missing wine, look at the mocktails in the first trimester recipes, and if you want a mid-afternoon energy boost flick through all the sections to find a muffin, flapjack or cookie recipe that takes your fancy. Enjoy your pregnancy and feel confident that you're meeting your baby's needs as well as satisfying your taste buds.

1 Healthy eating for pregnancy

What you eat during pregnancy will affect your baby's health for her entire life. This may seem daunting, but it actually means you have a great opportunity to set her on the right path before she's even born. This doesn't mean you need to obsess about every bite you take, as worrying isn't good for your baby either. If you're feeling nauseous and only eat toast for a day or two, there's no need to beat yourself up! Likewise, if you didn't eat the perfect diet before finding out you were pregnant, there really is no need to panic. But if you know your diet is far from ideal, try to start making small changes in the right direction. If you snack on fruit instead of biscuits you'll benefit now and your baby will grow up seeing this as the norm. Of course, you'll probably be trying to get her to eat more healthily for many years to come, but it is never going to be as easy as it is now to make sure she gets her greens.

Eating well now will also help *you* stay healthy and reduce the risk of developing problems such as gestational diabetes, raised blood pressure and piles. Dads-to-be aren't off the hook either. A good diet will make sure they're in peak condition, ready for the demands of fatherhood, and are around to enjoy being a dad for many years to come. Your baby will also benefit by being born into a household where healthy food is the norm.

Knowing which foods are healthy and safe can seem confusing at first, but it's not really that difficult. If you're worried your diet is nowhere near ideal at the moment, don't panic. Take it slowly. Gradually make small changes, replacing unhealthy choices with healthier ones. There are plenty of tasty foods that are good for you and your baby. Following the recipes and meal plans in this book will help your baby get off to a great start in life.

How your diet affects your baby

Quite simply, a woman who doesn't eat enough is likely to have a smaller and less healthy baby. You might think it would be possible to fatten the baby up after birth and get her doing just as well as the babies of well-nourished mothers, but that doesn't appear to be the case. Poor nutrition in the womb can permanently alter the structure of the heart, kidneys and other organs. Babies born with a birth weight at the lower end of the range are more likely to develop degenerative diseases, including obesity, heart disease and cancer.

However, eating lots of food while you're pregnant isn't the answer, as this is not the same as eating well. Overnutrition, as it is known, is a growing problem. It's just a different form of malnutrition. Scientists are discovering that overnutrition also results in irreversible differences in the way babies develop in the womb, leading to increased risks of obesity and type 2 diabetes.

What you need is a balanced diet, to ensure you get all the vitamins and minerals your baby needs. For example, you need to make sure you get enough iron, selenium and vitamin E. Iron deficiency can result in premature birth, low birth weight and pre-eclampsia, while good intakes of selenium and vitamin E have been found to reduce a baby's risk of developing asthma and eczema.

Clearly, it's not practical for you to take each individual nutrient and assess whether you're getting enough of it each day. However, it is possible to think about the broad food groups and try to eat from each one every day. If you have a variety of foods from each group, you can be pretty sure you'll be covered on most nutrients.

If you do skip a particular food group, then you should look more closely at the nutrients you might be missing out on and try to find alternatives. For example, if you don't have milk or milk products, like yogurt or cheese, you need other sources of calcium. Children whose mums have low calcium intakes have been found to have weaker bones. Milk and milk products are also the main source of vitamin B12, which is important for your baby's red blood cells and for iodine, which is needed for brain development. Researchers are making new discoveries all the time about how particular nutrients and phytonutrients affect a baby's development in the womb. In the past few years it has also become evident that a mother's diet can actually affect her baby's DNA, in terms of which genes are turned on and off. This in turn could have an impact on her baby's susceptibility to certain diseases or conditions, and be passed on to future generations.

What is a healthy diet for pregnancy

While you're pregnant it's important to eat as varied and healthy a diet as possible. You don't need any extra calories for the first two trimesters, and in the final trimester you only need about 200 calories more than usual. There are no particular foods that you absolutely must have, but if you eat foods from all the different groups your baby will get the nutrients she needs to grow and develop.

Fruit and vegetables

Aiming for at least five portions of fruit and vegetables a day is more important now than ever. They're packed with antioxidants, such as vitamin C and beta-carotene. These are important for the development of your baby's immune system and having a good intake can reduce the risk of your baby developing allergies. They're also important for your own health. Women eating more antioxidant-rich foods are less likely to develop pre-eclampsia.

Protein-rich foods

Protein provides the building blocks for growth, so it's essential for your baby. It is also vital for the development of the placenta and production of breast milk. Good sources include lean meat, chicken, fish, eggs, milk and dairy produce, and chickpeas, beans, lentils and other pulses.

Starchy carbohydrates

Foods such as rice, pasta, potatoes, breakfast cereals and bread provide carbohydrates, which are the main source of energy (or calories) in a healthy diet. If you choose unrefined versions, such as wholegrain cereals and bread and brown rice and pasta, you'll also get more vitamins and minerals – and more fibre, to help keep constipation at bay. These less refined foods also have a lower glycaemic index (GI); eating them will help stabilise your blood sugar levels and make it less likely that you'll put on too much weight (see p32).

Milk and dairy foods

Calcium is important for the growth of strong bones and teeth. Milk and dairy products, such as yogurt and cheese, are the main sources for most women. If you don't eat these, you should make sure you get enough calcium from other sources, such as fortified soya products, almonds and sesame seeds. As milk is also an important source of iodine, you'll also need to get this from other foods (p38).

Iron-rich foods

Iron is needed for healthy red blood cells. During pregnancy women are particularly prone to anaemia if they don't get enough. Meat and fish are good sources of iron, but we get most of our iron from breakfast cereals with added iron, and from foods such as bread, lentils, baked beans, peas and dried fruit.

Oily fish

Pregnant women are advised to eat two portions of fish a week. At least one of these should be oily fish, such as salmon or mackerel. These provide long-chain omega 3 fatty acids, which are important for brain and eye development (see p129). If you don't eat fish you can get long-chain omega 3s from supplements (p76).

Weight gain

Most of the weight women gain during pregnancy is due to their growing baby, the placenta and the amniotic fluid the baby is swimming in. In addition, your blood volume increases during pregnancy along with the tissue in your breasts and uterus. This explains why you might gain as much as two stone, but have a baby who weighs seven pounds. It is also quite normal and healthy for your body to lay down extra fat in preparation for breastfeeding.

However, eating for two doesn't mean eating double portions. If you eat whatever you fancy, you could end up putting on too much body fat. This can result in problems for both you and your baby and leave you with a couple of stone to lose once your baby is born.

Weight gain during pregnancy varies enormously and the right amount for you will depend on how much you weighed before becoming pregnant. Women who were overweight need to gain much less than those who were underweight in order to have a good pregnancy and a healthy baby. In the UK, there are no official recommendations about weight gain. However, in the USA women are given guidelines based on research into weight gains associated with the lowest risk of complications and the best chances of having a healthy baby.

BMI before pregnancy	Recommended weight gain	
Underweight, less than 18.5	12.5–18kg	2st to 2st 12lb
Healthy weight, 18.5–25	11.5–16kg	1st 11lb to 2st 7lb
Overweight, 25–30	7–11.5kg	1st 1lb to 1st 11lb
Obese, more than 30	5–9kg	11lb to 1st 6lb

Source: Kathleen M. Rasmussen and Ann L. Yaktine (eds), *Weight Gain During Pregnancy: Re-examining the guidelines*, Washington, DC: National Academies Press, 2009.

If you don't put on enough weight during pregnancy, your baby is more likely to be born prematurely and to have a low birth weight. This could result in long-term health problems for your baby. Putting on too much weight is just as much of a problem and is becoming increasingly common. This can result in women having raised blood pressure, pre-eclampsia and gestational diabetes, as well as making labour more difficult and increasing the likelihood of needing a caesarean delivery.

Research has found that women are more likely to gain a healthy amount of weight if they regularly stand on the scales and monitor how they're doing. Studies show that it helps to eat breakfast every day, have starchy foods at each meal and have plenty of fruit, vegetables and other fibre-rich foods. It's also important to have a low fat diet and avoid sugary drinks and snacks. In fact, a good diet for pregnancy really isn't that different to a balanced diet for general health.

Keeping active is important too. The NHS recommends at least 30 minutes of moderate exercise per day during pregnancy. This can include classes at your local gym or leisure centre, swimming or just brisk walking. As well as helping with weight gain, keeping active will make you feel healthier and less stressed and will lead to a better night's sleep. If you're struggling with your weight, make sure you talk to your doctor or midwife about your worries.

Foods and drinks to avoid

When you first became pregnant, you may have thought more about what to avoid than what is actually beneficial to eat. There are certainly enough media scare stories and ill-informed advice to make even the most level-headed woman worry. But it's important to sort the fact from the fiction and put things in perspective.

The table below shows the most up-to-date advice about which foods are considered high risk in pregnancy. You may find that other books or websites say you shouldn't eat peanuts or Stilton or that swordfish is fine in pregnancy, but this is outdated advice. The information below and in the rest of the book is based on current advice from the NHS, Department of Health, Food Standards Agency and National Institute for Health and Care Excellence (NICE). It may seem confusing and slightly ridiculous that the advice about what's safe and what's not changes. However, new research is constantly being carried out and new food problems emerge, so the advice changes based on the evidence available at any particular time.

The chances of getting food poisoning are very small, but you are more at risk of becoming ill during pregnancy because of changes to your immune system. Getting food poisoning during pregnancy can have devastating effects and can result in miscarriage, or disability for your baby.

This may seem like a long list but it will soon become second nature, and it's good to know that there are plenty of alternatives you can enjoy without worrying.

What to avoid	Why?	What's safe?
Soft mould-ripened cheeses (e.g. Brie, Camembert, chèvre) and soft blue cheeses (e.g. Danish blue, St Agur).	Risk of listeria, whether the cheese is made from pasteurised or unpasteurised milk. Listeria can result in miscarriage, stillbirth and severe illness in newborn babies.	Hard cheeses (e.g. Cheddar, Parmesan), semi-hard cheeses (e.g. Leerdammer, Edam) and soft cheeses made from pasteurised milk (e.g. cottage cheese, cream cheese, feta, mozzarella, ricotta). Also see p29 and p83.
Raw and partially cooked eggs (e.g. soft-boiled eggs, fried eggs with a runny yolk, home-made mousse, mayonnaise and ice cream).	Salmonella may be present and although it wouldn't cross the placenta and directly affect the baby, it can cause a high temperature and severe vomiting, which could be harmful (p41).	Eggs cooked until both the white and yolk are solid. Also, products made with cooked eggs (e.g. cakes, biscuits) or pasteurised egg (e.g. supermarket-bought mayonnaise or custard). Also see p120.
Unpasteurised milk (e.g. raw cows', goats' and sheep's milk) and milk products (e.g. yogurt or cream made with unpasteurised milk).	It may contain salmonella, E. coli and Brucella, which could all result in severe food poisoning.	Pasteurised, UHT or powdered milk and products such as yogurt and cream sold in supermarkets.
Liver, liver products (e.g. liver pâté, liver sausage) and cod liver oil supplements.	These contain high levels of retinol, which is a form of vitamin A. Very high intakes are associated with birth defects.	Foods high in beta-carotene, the other form of vitamin A, such as carrots (see p70).
Raw and undercooked meat (e.g. rare steak) including cold cured meat (e.g. salami, chorizo, Parma ham).	These may contain microscopic parasites that cause toxoplasmosis, which can result in miscarriage and severe birth defects.	Meat without any traces of pinkness. Cured meats that have been frozen and those in cooked dishes such as chorizo in soup.

Continued over page

My Pregnancy Recipes and Meal Planner

Continued from overleaf

What to avoid	Why?	What's safe?
Shark, swordfish and marlin.	These fish may contain high levels of mercury, which can damage an unborn baby's nervous system.	Any other fish, see below for amounts.
Too much oily fish (e.g. salmon, mackerel, sardines).	These contain pollutants that could be harmful in large amounts.	Up to two portions of oily fish a week is considered beneficial (see p129). You can eat as many portions of most white fish as you like (e.g. cod, coley, haddock). Also see p90.
Too much tuna.	May contain mercury and pollutants.	Up to two portions of fresh tuna or four tins a week.
Raw or undercooked shellfish (e.g. oysters, prawns, mussels).	May be contaminated with bacteria, viruses and toxins.	Prawns in hot dishes such as fish pie. Shellfish that has been cooked and chilled carefully.
Raw bean sprouts.	Salmonella, E. coli and other bacteria may be present and could cause food poisoning.	Bean sprouts that are thoroughly cooked in a hot dish such as a stir-fry.
Pâté (e.g. liver pâté, salmon pâté, mushroom pâté).	Risk of listeria.	Home-made pâté made following good hygiene rules (e.g. sardine pâté on p164).
Too much coffee, tea or other drinks containing caffeine.	High intakes are associated with miscarriage and low birth weight.	Up to 200mg per day is considered safe. A mug of instant coffee contains about 100mg and a mug of tea about 75mg of caffeine.
Alcohol.	Risk of miscarriage and birth defects (see p55).	No amount of alcohol has been shown to be safe in pregnancy. If you choose to drink, don't have more than 1 or 2 units once or twice a week.

While breastfeeding, you still need to be careful about how much caffeine and alcohol you drink as these substances pass into your breast milk. However, you can go back to eating soft-boiled eggs and any cheese you fancy (p149).

Food hygiene

As well as avoiding certain foods, you need to be particularly careful about food hygiene while you're pregnant.

- Always wash your hands before cooking or eating.
- Make sure kitchen work surfaces are clean and pet-free.
- Check your fridge is really below 5°C and your freezer below −17°C.
- Clean your fridge, never put anything in it that is uncovered and make sure raw meat is at the bottom so that it can't drip onto other foods.
- Wash all fruit and vegetables, even those labelled as 'washed and ready to eat' (p74).
- Don't eat anything after its 'use by' date, even if it looks and smells ok.
- Cool leftovers and get them in the fridge within an hour of cooking. Then eat them within 24 hours.
- Make sure hot foods are piping hot, right through to the middle, especially foods cooked in the microwave, ready meals and pies.

Supplements

There are some supplements that every pregnant woman should take, as research has shown they have clear benefits

> The Department of Health advises all women to take:
> - 400µg (micrograms) of folic acid per day before conception and for the first 12 weeks of pregnancy
> - 10µg of vitamin D per day throughout pregnancy and while breastfeeding.

Taking a folic acid supplement reduces your risk of having a baby with a neural tube defect (NTD) such as spina bifida or anencephaly. Most women should take 400µg, but if you are diabetic or have a family history of NTDs, then a higher dose may be recommended. It is best to ask your doctor or midwife for advice. Vitamin D deficiency is fairly common, affecting about one woman in three. Severe deficiency during pregnancy can result in babies suffering from seizures in the first few months of life and long-term bone disease (p21).

Many women choose to take a multivitamin and mineral supplement during pregnancy. If you have a healthy diet, these are not really necessary. However, they are a good idea for anyone who is diabetic or expecting twins and those with a limited diet, for example those on dairy-free diets or vegans. If you don't eat oily fish, then a supplement containing long-chain omega 3 fatty acids may also be a good idea (see p75).

If you decide to take supplements, make sure they specifically say that they are suitable for pregnant or breastfeeding women. Vitamin A supplements and any multivitamins containing vitamin A are not suitable for pregnancy as they can cause developmental problems. Also, bear in mind that while foods high in certain nutrients, such as antioxidants, have been found to be beneficial in pregnancy, this hasn't always been the case when the same nutrients are given as supplements. Indeed, these have sometimes been seen to have a detrimental effect – taking supplements isn't a quick fix for eating badly (see p80).

Recipes in this book

The recipes in this book are designed with pregnancy and breastfeeding in mind, but they are suitable for anyone who wants to eat healthily. They are generally low in fat, saturated fat and salt, and rich in antioxidants, and so are ideal for anyone wanting to maintain a healthy weight and long-term health. They can be enjoyed by dads-to-be and friends and family too. You can adjust the recipes according to your own needs – for example, if you're putting on too much weight then use reduced fat cheese rather than full fat.

If you already have children, hopefully they will enjoy these recipes as well. Most of the main meals are for two adults, but some are for four people. This is particularly the case for soups, where it is almost easier to make more, and stews, that take longer to cook. These dishes freeze well, so it makes sense to prepare extra that can be used another day.

If you are cooking for more, you can obviously just double up on ingredients. The number of portions is only approximate anyway, as pregnancy can make you ravenously hungry or have hardly any appetite at all.

The recipes are organised by trimester, with a separate section for breastfeeding mums, but there's no reason you shouldn't flick through and use recipes from different sections. A recipe may be particularly suited to early pregnancy because it contains ginger to help with morning sickness, but the nutrients are just as important later on in pregnancy.

Author's recipe notes

- Although the instructions for each recipe don't mention **washing fruit and vegetables**, it is always important to do this (p74).
- An approximate **preparation time** is given for each recipe. A separate cooking time is also given for dishes that can be left to simmer or bake while you get on with other things. If foods need watching while they cook or other ingredients need to be prepared, then the cooking time is included in the overall preparation time.
- Where tablespoon (tbsp) or teaspoon (tsp) quantities are given, these should be level spoonfuls, unless otherwise stated.
- Medium eggs have been used when creating these recipes, but if you use large eggs the recipes will still work fine.
- Rapeseed oil is used in many recipes to make them healthier (p52). If you substitute butter or margarine for oil when baking, use 45g butter or margarine in place of 50ml rapeseed oil.

Abbreviations used

°C – degrees centigrade

cm – centimetres

°F – degrees Fahrenheit

g – grams

ml – millilitres

mm – millimetres

tbsp – tablespoon (approx. 15g/15ml)

tsp – teaspoon (approx. 5g/5ml)

Conversion chart

We have used metric measurements throughout the book. Should you want to convert the measurements to imperial, here is a rough guide.

Metric	Imperial
Grams (g)	Ounces (oz)
25g	1oz
50g	2oz
100g	3½oz
150g	5oz
Millilitres (ml)	Fluid ounces (fl oz)
50ml	1¾fl oz
100ml	3½fl oz
150ml	5fl oz
Centimetres (cm)	Inches
2.5cm	1 inch

2 The first trimester

Finding out you're pregnant can be both exciting and daunting. In many ways this first trimester is the most difficult as you don't have a bump yet and other people probably don't know you're having a baby. At the same time you may be feeling a bit tired and emotional. Even if you're not suffering from morning sickness you're probably not quite your normal self.

Some women find taste changes are the first sign of pregnancy. It may be that they go off coffee or can't stop thinking about a juicy steak. For every woman it's different! While some changes in taste are beneficial, going off alcohol for example, others, like craving salt and vinegar crisps, are definitely not. Contrary to popular belief, there's no evidence that cravings are linked to what your body or your baby needs. So while it's fine to have a few fruit pastilles, if that's what you're craving, you certainly don't *need* to eat a packet every day. If you're hankering after sugary or salty snacks, it's better if you can find a healthier alternative. For example, if you want something sour or tangy, try fresh fruit, lemon yogurt (p46) or marmalade flapjacks (p52). That way, you and your baby will also get beneficial nutrients.

If you are craving chalk, mud or any other non-foods, these particularly unusual taste changes could be a sign of iron deficiency, so it's a good idea to have your iron levels tested as soon as possible. It might also be wise to increase your iron intake just in case (see p110).

Morning sickness is a problem for eight out of 10 women, and if you're one of them it will inevitably affect what you eat. Those suffering from severe morning sickness, with frequent vomiting, need medical help in order to protect the baby. But in most cases it's very unlikely to affect your baby's health. In fact, morning sickness appears to be a positive sign, as it shows your hormones are changing as they should. It also helps to protect your baby, by forcing you to rest and take care of yourself. If you're hardly eating anything, it's much more likely that *you* will suffer, rather than your baby, so try not to worry. Eat as healthily as possible, but if all you can manage is dry toast or biscuits, then have that until you're feeling better. Most women find that morning sickness subsides by the end of the first trimester, and by week 14 symptoms usually disappear completely.

Although morning sickness can occur at any time of day, it's often worse in the morning when blood sugar levels are low. So eating breakfast can help. Eating little and often throughout the day will also help to keep blood sugar levels more stable. You may be tempted to reach for a quick sugar fix, but research has shown that women who have more sugar are more likely to suffer from nausea. Instead, it's better to eat smaller meals and try some of the other strategies listed below.

How to relieve morning sickness

- Avoid any triggers, such as particular smells or foods.
- Eat little and often to keep blood sugar levels stable.
- Eat ginger (see p50).
- Rest as much as possible, as tiredness makes symptoms worse.
- Drink plenty of fluids, as dehydration can make you feel worse.
- Try a complementary therapy, such as acupressure wristbands, acupuncture, homeopathy or aromatherapy.
- Go outside for some fresh air or find something to distract you.

Some women find they prefer to eat bland foods that don't have a strong smell or taste and they go off anything fried or spicy. If this is the case, you can try eating light meals such as chicken noodle soup (p23) and baked fish with couscous (p37). You might also enjoy the recipes containing ginger, which has long been known to reduce the symptoms of nausea. You can have ginger with your breakfast, lunch or dinner or have it in snacks if that suits you better (see p50).

How to ginger up your day

- A soup (see pp22 and 23) or main course with added ginger (see pp33, 36, 37, 38 and 40)
- Ginger biscuits and cookies (see pp49 and 50)
- Ginger drinks (see pp54 and 55)
- Ginger sweets

While going off your food is common in early pregnancy, so is feeling incredibly hungry. It's also quite normal to feel nauseous and hungry at the same time. Many women find they feel sick if they don't eat. Although it may seem strange that you want to eat more when your baby is no bigger than a grape, your body is already undergoing lots of changes. Your blood volume is increasing, the placenta is forming and, as you've probably noticed, extra breast tissue is being formed. While hormonal changes are responsible for an increase in appetite, it's up to you what you do about it. If you're underweight or fairly slim, then it's a good idea to eat more, but if you're overweight then try not to use pregnancy as an excuse for eating too much. Either way, try to stick to healthy meals and snacks which will provide essential nutrients. Whenever possible, eat foods with a low glycaemic index (GI), as these will help stabilise your blood sugar levels and keep hunger at bay for longer (p32).

Healthy snacks to keep nausea and hunger at bay

- A banana or other fresh fruit
- A pot of yogurt
- Rice cakes with marmite or peanut butter
- A bowl of muesli or other wholegrain breakfast cereal
- Oatcakes with reduced fat cream cheese
- Some chicken or lentil soup
- A small portion of unsalted nuts or mixed nuts and dried fruit
- Snacks containing oats, such as oat and raisin cookies (p51) or marmalade flapjacks (p52)
- Anything containing ginger, including triple ginger cookies (p49)

As your body is adapting to pregnancy you may notice more bloating, wind, constipation or just general abdominal discomfort. This is because your digestive system is starting to slow down so you can absorb extra nutrients from the food you eat. Having a good fibre intake can help with constipation, along with drinking plenty of fluids and keeping physically active. Increasing your fluid intake is also beneficial if you are suffering from nausea or headaches.

Eating as healthily as possible at this stage of pregnancy will get your baby off to a good start. However, if you're not feeling well, don't get stressed about what you think you should be doing. Certainly don't worry about what you ate before you knew you were pregnant or any alcohol you drank. The important part is that from now on you can avoid the foods and drinks that could cause problems (p7) and make other healthy choices. Skipping alcohol without broadcasting your pregnancy can be a problem but there are plenty of tactics you can use.

Top tactics for avoiding alcohol

- Say you're on antibiotics for a bladder infection or another problem that people won't want to discuss.
- Explain you're on a fasting day for the 5:2 diet, you're on a detox, or just trying to lose some weight.
- Drive to the pub or restaurant.
- Order a non-alcohol version of your usual drink when you go to the bar, such as a mocktail, alcohol-free lager, coke without the rum, or tonic without the gin.
- Offer to hold the kitty and go up to the bar if you're with a group.
- Tell just one good friend that you're pregnant, then he or she will know what you really want when you ask for your usual.
- Claim to have given up alcohol for January, Lent or in preparation for Christmas or a big occasion.
- Say you're recovering from an awful hangover.
- Tell friends you've got an early start in the morning.
- Accept a drink if it's unavoidable but don't actually drink it – nurse it, leave it somewhere, swap it with a friend or tip it away.

You should also start taking supplements now if you haven't already (p9). Eat nutritious foods when you can, and, as you feel better, eat more of them. The recipes in this section are really designed to make it as easy as possible for you to eat well. In addition to recipes for healthy snacking and combating morning sickness, there are fish recipes for those who don't usually eat fish, or are put off by the smell of it cooking, and there's beef stew (p45) and Osborne pudding (p48) for when your hormones are playing havoc and you need comfort food.

Breakfasts

Cinnamon and banana porridge

Sachets of quick oats are convenient but they only make small portions and contain 25% sugar, which means you're hungry by mid-morning if not before. This breakfast is just as easy to prepare (only 3 minutes in the microwave), tastier, cheaper, healthier and it will keep you going until lunchtime.

50g porridge oats
¼ tsp cinnamon plus extra for sprinkling
150ml (150g) milk
150ml (150g) water
1 tsp demerara sugar or honey
1 banana

Preparation time: 1 minute plus 3 minutes in the microwave.
Equipment: 1 bowl.
Storage: Eat straightaway.
Servings: 1.

- Place the oats, cinnamon, milk and water in a large bowl. You can either use a measuring jug or weigh the liquid on the scales.
- Microwave for 2 minutes then stir and microwave for another 1 minute.
- Stir, sprinkle with the sugar and slice the banana on top. You might like to add a little cold milk around the edge of the bowl too.

Tips

- Make sure your bowl is big enough as the porridge will bubble up while it's cooking. A large, fairly deep soup bowl is better than a shallow cereal bowl.
- If you prefer you can make the porridge with all milk or all water, rather than half and half.
- Instead of banana you can put fresh berries on top or sprinkle on a few nuts or seeds. You could also try mixing some dried fruit with the oats before cooking. Sultanas or chopped dried apricots work well.

Why you should eat breakfast

Breakfast eaters are more likely to get all the nutrients they need than those who skip it. A study of 600 pregnant women in Pittsburgh, USA, found that those who regularly ate breakfast cereals had higher intakes of calcium, folate, iron, zinc and vitamins A, C, D and E. You might think that those who skip breakfast make up for it later in the day, but the tendency is to reach for snack foods which are high in sugar and fat and low in essential vitamins and minerals. Many breakfast cereals have the added advantage of being fortified with vitamins and iron, but the Pittsburgh study found that even women eating unfortified cereals, such as muesli, were less likely to be deficient in these key nutrients, which are vital for healthy fetal and placental development.

Pear and ginger breakfast crumble

This makes a great breakfast with natural yogurt – it's a cross between a traditional fruit crumble and granola cereal. It has ginger to help keep morning sickness at bay or revive you if you wake up feeling less than glowing, and oats to help stabilise blood sugar levels, which will also help to combat nausea.

Topping
100g oats
50g wholemeal flour
2 tbsp honey
50ml rapeseed oil
50g crystallised ginger

Filling
4 large pears
1 tbsp lemon juice
1 tbsp wholemeal flour
2 tsp ground ginger

To serve
natural yogurt

Preparation time: 15 minutes plus 25 minutes baking.
Equipment: 1 mixing bowl and 1 ovenproof dish.
Storage: Fridge for 1–2 days or freeze.

Servings: 4.

- Preheat the oven to 200°C (180°C fan)/400°F/gas mark 6.
- In the mixing bowl, stir together all the ingredients for the topping. If the ginger is in large chunks you may want to break them up or chop them into pea-sized pieces.
- Quarter the pears, then peel and core them and cut into chunks.
- Put the pear pieces in the ovenproof dish, sprinkle the lemon juice over the top and stir. Mix the extra spoonful of flour with the ground ginger and stir in to coat the chunks of pear.
- Scatter the topping over the pears and place in the oven for 25 minutes until nicely browned.
- Eat cold, or warm it up in the microwave, and serve with a few spoonfuls of yogurt.

Tips

- To make it even more nutritious you can add some chopped nuts, such as pecans, to the topping mixture.
- Apples work well in this too or use a mixture of apples and pears. You can also use rhubarb, but either cook it first or use the tinned variety.

Made-to-measure muesli

Home-made muesli, with no added sugar or flavourings, tastes wonderful and takes only minutes to prepare. But the best thing about it is you can make it exactly as you like. Keep it simple with raisins, add apricots for extra iron and a zestier flavour, or prunes, if you feel the need. If you find whole Brazil nuts a bit too much first thing in the morning you can chop them up or use other nuts instead. This basic recipe gives you a rough guide to quantities, then you can take it from there.

200g porridge oats
75g apricots
50g prunes
30g flaked almonds
50g Brazil nuts
50g mixed seeds

Preparation time: 10 minutes.
Equipment: An airtight container.

Storage: Store in airtight container for several weeks.
Servings: 10.

- Chop the apricots, prunes and Brazil nuts.
- Combine all the ingredients in the container.

Tips

- If you're using dried fruit that is 'ready to eat', it may say it should be stored in the fridge, in which case you can keep the whole container of muesli in the fridge.
- Other fruits you can try include sultanas, raisins, dates and figs.
- Brazil nuts are particularly good because they are very rich in selenium (p143) but you can also use hazelnuts, walnuts, cashews or pecans.
- Eating your muesli with a handful of bran flakes will increase your intake of insoluble fibre, also known as roughage, and your iron and B vitamin intake (if you choose a brand of flakes with these added).
- Serve with a dollop of yogurt and a handful of fresh or defrosted frozen berries for an even better antioxidant boost.

Banana bread

If you wake up craving cake this is ideal – likewise if you can't face breakfast but need something mid-morning to keep you going. It's packed with bananas instead of sugar, has eggs and nuts for extra protein and it's made with wholemeal flour to boost your fibre intake and supply your baby with extra micronutrients.

5 small ripe bananas (about 450g including skin)
100ml (100g) rapeseed oil plus extra for greasing
2 eggs
175g wholemeal flour
75g oats
2 tsp baking powder
1 tsp ground mixed spice
½ tsp bicarbonate of soda
50g chopped walnuts

Preparation time: 15 minutes plus 45 minutes baking.
Equipment: 1 mixing bowl, 1 measuring jug and a 2lb loaf tin (about 22cm x 11cm internally).

Storage: Airtight container for a few days or freeze.
Servings: 1 loaf.

- Preheat the oven to 180°C (160°C fan)/350°F/gas mark 4. Grease the loaf tin and line with greaseproof paper.
- Measure the oil into a jug then crack the eggs into the oil and beat lightly.
- Peel the bananas, slice into the bowl and mash with a potato masher or fork.
- Pour the egg mixture into the bowl with the mashed bananas and combine with a fork.
- Stir in the flour, oats, baking powder, mixed spice and bicarbonate of soda, then fold in the walnuts.
- Pour the mixture into the prepared tin, smooth over and bake for about 45–50 minutes until a skewer inserted in the centre comes out dry.
- Leave to cool for 5–10 minutes before removing from the tin and peeling off the greaseproof paper, then leave on a cooling rack until completely cool.

Tip

- The riper your bananas the sweeter this will taste, so if they're not ripe you can add some honey or sugar to the recipe, or just wait until they ripen.

Why you should have vitamin D – the sunshine vitamin

'Vitamin D is an unusual vitamin as our bodies can make it from the action of sunlight on our skin. In the UK, however, we can only do this during the summer and research suggests that many people have low levels of vitamin D. Vitamin D controls the absorption of calcium from our food and helps regulate calcium levels in the blood. Insufficient vitamin D in pregnancy and infancy causes rickets in children. A condition causing bone pain called osteomalacia can occur in adults too. Therefore the Department of Health recommends that pregnant and breastfeeding women take a daily supplement containing 10 micrograms. This is particularly important if you have a darker skin or cover up for religious reasons. You can make sure that you eat some vitamin D rich foods too. These include fortified breakfast cereals, oily fish, fortified margarine and eggs.'

Dr Gail Rees, Associate Professor of Human Nutrition, Plymouth University

Lunches, dinners and sides

Creamy butternut squash and red pepper soup

This delicious soup is low in fat but tasty and comforting, making it easy to reach the 5-a-day target. It also contains ginger to help you fight off morning sickness.

1 tbsp olive oil
1 onion
1 red pepper
1 butternut squash
1–2 tsp grated fresh root ginger
¼ tsp sweet paprika
500ml stock
1 tbsp cream cheese

To serve
salt and pepper
natural yogurt (optional)
fresh chives (optional)

Preparation time: 15 minutes plus 20 minutes simmering.
Equipment: 1 pan and a stick blender.
Storage: Fridge for 24 hours or freeze.
Servings: 3–4.

- Peel and dice the onion. Heat the oil in the pan then add the onion and sweat over a low heat for 2–3 minutes with the lid on.
- Cut the pepper in half, remove the seeds, wash and dice.
- Cut the squash in half lengthways, remove the seeds and skin and chop into 2cm chunks.
- Add the pepper, squash, grated ginger and sweet paprika to the pan and cook for a few minutes more.
- Add the stock, bring to the boil and simmer with the lid on for 20 minutes until the vegetables are tender.
- Remove from the heat, add the cream cheese and whiz with a stick blender until completely smooth.

- Add salt and pepper to taste, and, if you like, serve topped with a spoonful of yogurt and a few chopped chives.

Why you should eat more vegetables

Vegetables are packed with vitamins and minerals, including beta-carotene for your baby's eye development and vitamin C for healthy new cells. They also provide potassium to help control your blood pressure and fibre to keep constipation at bay. If you're struggling to eat good healthy meals, then soups are a great way to boost your intake. They're generally a healthier alternative to fruit juices, as they contain less sugar and have a lower glycaemic index (GI), so they help keep your blood sugar levels stable. Try to eat as wide a variety of vegetables as possible, including dark green, deep yellow, orange, red and purple varieties, then you'll benefit from the wide range of beneficial phytochemicals the different types contain.

Chicken noodle soup

A real feel-good meal. This light and tasty broth with chicken, vegetables and noodles makes a great lunch or light supper.

2 spring onions
1 tsp rapeseed oil
1 clove garlic
1 tsp grated fresh root ginger
1 chicken breast
1 litre stock
1 large carrot
2 handfuls shredded cabbage or pak choi
4 mushrooms
2 tsp soya sauce
100g noodles, dried or straight to wok

Preparation time: 30 minutes.
Equipment: 1 large pan with a lid.
Storage: Fridge for 24 hours.
Servings: 2.

- Slice the spring onions. Heat the oil in the pan and sauté the onions for 2 minutes. Add the crushed garlic and ginger and cook for another minute.

- Cut the chicken breast in half then place it in the pan. Cover with the stock then bring to the boil and simmer for 20 minutes with the lid on.
- Meanwhile, peel the carrot and slice into matchstick-sized pieces. Slice the mushrooms.
- When the chicken is cooked, take it out of the pan using two forks and put it on a plate. Put the vegetables and soya sauce into the pan and bring back to the boil then simmer for 1–2 minutes.
- Meanwhile, using the forks, shred the chicken into bite-sized pieces.
- Return the chicken to the pan, along with the noodles and stir. Continue cooking until the noodles are ready.

Tips

- You can use any kind of noodles you like – dried egg noodles, thin vermicelli rice noodles, straight to wok noodles or instant noodles (just throw away the sachet of flavouring they come with).
- To make a vegetarian version you can use tofu instead of chicken.
- Try a fish version by chopping white fish into bite-sized pieces and adding at the same time as the noodles.

Spinach and feta frittata

Frittatas are really just fancy omelettes with extra ingredients. This one is very easy to make and the spinach goes perfectly with salty feta.

2 tsp olive oil or rapeseed oil
½ small onion
90g frozen chopped spinach or fresh if preferred
8 cherry tomatoes
3 eggs
40g feta cheese
black pepper

Preparation time: 15 minutes.
Equipment: 1 frying pan (about 24cm diameter).
Storage: Fridge for up to 24 hours.
Servings: 2.

- Put the spinach in the microwave for 2 minutes.
- Peel and finely slice the onion.
- Heat the oil in the frying pan and fry the onion for 2–3 minutes.

- Press the spinach with the back of a spoon or fork and drain away as much liquid as possible.
- Add the spinach to the pan along with the cherry tomatoes, cut in half.
- While the vegetables are cooking, lightly beat the eggs.
- Add the eggs to the pan and spread out the ingredients so that they're roughly even.
- While the frittata is cooking, crumble the feta cheese over the top and add a good sprinkle of black pepper.
- Cook over a medium heat for 5 minutes, until the sides are set but the top is still runny. Run a spatula around the edge of the pan to separate the cooked eggs from the pan but don't stir the mixture.
- Place under the grill for a couple of minutes, until it is completely set and the top is nicely browned, then transfer to a plate and cut into wedges.

Courgette, ricotta and basil frittata

This light Mediterranean dish is delicious either warm with new potatoes and green beans or cold with bread and salad.

1 large courgette
1 tsp olive oil
4 eggs
1 tbsp grated Parmesan or pecorino cheese
100g ricotta
1 tbsp chopped fresh basil or ½ tsp dried basil
black pepper

Preparation time: 15 minutes.
Equipment: 1 frying pan.
Storage: Fridge for 24 hours.
Servings: 2.

- Wash the courgette, cut off the ends, slice in half lengthways then slice thinly.
- Heat the oil in a frying pan and fry the courgette for about 5 minutes, until lightly browned.
- Beat the eggs together with the ricotta, grated cheese, basil and some black pepper.
- Pour the egg mixture over the cooked courgettes and cook over a medium heat for 5 minutes, until the bottom is browned but the top is still runny.

Run a spatula around the edge of the pan to separate the cooked eggs from the pan but don't stir the mixture.

- Place under the grill for a couple of minutes, until it is completely set and the top is nicely browned, then transfer to a plate and cut into wedges.

Why you shouldn't eat runny eggs

Unless eggs are cooked until both the white and the yolk are solid, there is a risk of food poisoning from salmonella bacteria. This is one of the most common forms of food poisoning and can result in abdominal pain, diarrhoea and a fever. When you buy eggs, it's best to choose ones with the British Lion Quality stamp, store them in the fridge and eat them before the 'use by' date. You need to be especially careful when eating out, as the FSA has found caterers don't always follow these guidelines. You should also avoid foods made with raw or partially cooked eggs, such as home-made mayonnaise, custard, carbonara sauce, ice cream or mousse.

Peanut butter houmous

This is incredibly easy to make and uses peanut butter instead of tahini, which is easier to get hold of and you're more likely to use the rest of the jar. It's also very tasty and will help satisfy peanut cravings.

1 x 400g tin chickpeas
2 tbsp peanut butter (smooth or crunchy)
1 tbsp lemon juice
½ tsp ground cumin
1 tbsp sesame or olive oil or a mixture
3 tbsp natural yogurt (use avocado or water instead for a dairy-free version)
½–1 clove garlic (optional)
salt and freshly ground black pepper

Preparation time: 5 minutes.
Equipment: 1 blender or bowl and a stick blender.
Storage: Fridge for 2 days or freeze.
Servings: 2–4.

- Drain the chickpeas and place in the blender or bowl with the rest of the ingredients, apart from the salt and pepper.

- Blend until smooth.
- Taste and add salt and pepper or more lemon juice according to taste.

Tip

- Other ingredients you might like to add include sweet chilli sauce, caramelised onion chutney, sun-dried tomatoes, pickled roast red pepper, olives or beetroot.

Smoked mackerel pâté

Smoked mackerel is combined with peppery horseradish and tangy lemon in this easy pâté. If the smell of fish cooking is off-putting just now, then this is an ideal alternative.

2 smoked mackerel fillets
75g crème fraîche
50g cream cheese (e.g. Philadelphia)
1 tbsp creamed horseradish
zest of ½ a lemon
2 tsp lemon juice
black pepper
3 spring onions (optional)

Preparation time: 10 minutes.
Equipment: 1 bowl and a blender (optional).
Storage: Fridge for 24 hours.
Servings: 2 for lunch or 4 as a starter.

- Carefully peel the skin off the mackerel.
- Put the fish in the bowl and flake with a fork. Then add the remaining ingredients and mash together. Alternatively, put all the ingredients in a blender to produce a smoother pâté.
- Thinly slice the spring onion and scatter on top.

Tips

- You can use regular crème fraîche or cream cheese or reduced fat versions. If you use whole-fat versions of both, however, the pâté can end up tasting a bit too creamy.
- This tastes good with wholemeal toast or in a baked potato.
- Serve with watercress and beetroot salad (p76) for a good contrast in flavours.

Tastes and smells!

Many women notice a heightened sense of smell and taste when they're pregnant. A whiff of aftershave or the taste of meat can leave them feeling decidedly queasy. Increased levels of the hormone oestrogen are thought to be responsible for this and it could be nature's way of ensuring they avoid substances that could be harmful to their growing baby, such as cigarette smoke or alcohol. Why some women go off the smell of vegetables or their husband is more of a mystery! If you find certain tastes or smells make you feel more nauseous, then simply avoid them for now, open the window, eat more cold foods or ask someone else to cook. As pregnancy progresses you'll find things calm down.

Stuffed peppers with feta and olives

Have these tasty peppers with some bread and a mixed salad for lunch or as a side dish with fish or chicken.

2 peppers (red, yellow, green or orange)
2 tsp olive oil
salt and freshly ground black pepper
2 shallots
2–3 mushrooms
1 clove garlic
75g couscous
150ml boiling water
50g feta cheese
2 tbsp black olives
few chopped basil leaves

Preparation time: 20 minutes plus 20 minutes baking.
Equipment: 1 small frying pan and 1 baking tray.
Storage: Fridge for 1–2 days
Servings: 2 for lunch or 4 as a side dish.

- Cut the peppers in half lengthways across the stalk. Remove the stalk and seeds and rinse.
- Preheat the oven to 200°C (180°C fan)/400°F/gas mark 6.
- Place the peppers cut side up on a plate, drizzle with 1 teaspoon of oil and sprinkle with salt and pepper. Microwave on full power for 5 minutes.
- Meanwhile finely dice the shallots and dice the mushrooms.

- Heat the second teaspoon of oil in a small frying pan and fry the shallots, mushrooms and crushed garlic for a few minutes.
- Turn off the heat, then add the couscous and 150ml of boiling water and leave for a few minutes.
- Dice the feta cheese and roughly chop the black olives and basil, then stir into the couscous.
- Place the pepper halves on a baking tray, fill with the couscous mixture and bake for 20 minutes.

Tip

- Before serving, you may like to drizzle some extra olive oil on top or add a squeeze of lemon juice.

Why you shouldn't eat soft cheeses

You've probably been told to avoid soft and blue cheeses, but you may not know which ones are actually dangerous and why. Soft mould-ripened cheeses such as Brie, Camembert or any others with a soft white rind should be avoided. These have a high moisture content and eating them can result in food poisoning with listeria, whether they're made from pasteurised or unpasteurised milk. You should also avoid soft blue cheeses, such as Saint Agur and dolcelatte. However, feta and other 'Greek-style' cheeses that you buy in the UK are fine to eat, as are hard cheeses such as Cheddar and Edam, and soft cheeses like cream cheese, cottage cheese and ricotta. See also p83.

Aubergine and bean burgers

These bean burgers have a great flavour and texture and make a healthy alternative to regular burgers. They go well in a bread roll with salad, or have them with pasta and tomato sauce.

4 tsp rapeseed oil
1 small onion
1 aubergine
1 clove garlic
1 x 400g tin kidney beans
50g oats
1 tbsp tomato puree
1 tbsp chopped fresh basil or ½ tsp dried basil
1 egg
flour for dusting

Preparation time: 20 minutes plus 30 minutes in the fridge and 15 minutes cooking.
Equipment: 1 large pan and 1 frying pan.
Storage: Fridge for 24 hours or freeze.
Servings: 8 burgers (adults may want 1 or 2).

- Peel and finely dice the onion. Wash the aubergine and dice into 1cm cubes.
- Heat 2 teaspoons of oil in a pan, then sauté the onion, aubergine and crushed garlic for about 10 minutes until very soft. Remove from the heat.
- Drain the kidney beans and rinse, then add them to the aubergine mixture and mash with a potato masher.
- Add the oats, tomato puree, basil and egg to the pan and stir well.
- Shape the mixture into burgers using floured hands. Put the burgers on a plate and place them in the fridge for 30 minutes, or longer if you like, so that the mixture can bind together.
- To cook the burgers, heat 2 teaspoons of oil in a frying pan, then cook on a medium heat for about 15 minutes, turning once halfway through.

Why you should eat less meat and more vegetarian meals

In the past, meat was thought to be the best source of protein a person could get, but mounting evidence suggests that many people are eating too much red meat and processed meats, such as bacon and ham, and that they would benefit from having more vegetarian foods. According to the World Cancer Research Fund (WRCF), there is strong evidence that eating a lot of red meat is a cause of bowel cancer. Several studies have shown that vegetarians are less likely to get bowel or other types of cancer. The WRCF recommends substituting red meat with chicken or fish on some days and even trying to make every other evening meal completely meat free, having Quorn, lentils or beans instead. Kidney beans are especially great during pregnancy as they are high in soluble and insoluble fibre as well as providing iron and folate.

Baked lentil and ricotta 'meatballs'

These make a great supper with pasta and tomato sauce and you can have leftovers for lunch in warm pitta bread with some salad and yogurt.

1 x 400g tin green lentils (about 230g drained lentils)
1 egg
100g ricotta
1 tbsp (15g) Parmesan or other Italian hard cheese
1 clove garlic
40g wholemeal breadcrumbs
½ tsp paprika
1 tsp mixed herbs
2 tsp rapeseed oil

Preparation time: 10 minutes plus 30 minutes in the fridge and 25 minutes baking.
Equipment: 1 mixing bowl and 1 baking tray.
Storage: Fridge for 24 hours or freeze.
Servings: 12 meatballs.

- Drain the tinned lentils well, to remove as much water as possible, then transfer to a mixing bowl.
- Stir in the egg, ricotta, grated Parmesan, crushed garlic, breadcrumbs, paprika and herbs.
- Stir the mixture really well, then cover the bowl with cling film and put it in the fridge for 30 minutes, or longer if you like.
- Preheat the oven to 200°C (180°C fan)/400°F/gas mark 6.
- Cover the baking tray with a sheet of greaseproof paper and brush with one teaspoon of oil.
- Take a golf ball-sized piece of the lentil mixture, roll into a ball and place on the baking tray. When you have 12 meatballs, brush them with the remaining oil.
- Place in the oven for 25 minutes, turning over halfway through.

Fusilli with lentils and feta

Perfect when you're feeling tired but ravenously hungry. Although there are some cheeses that you can't eat now, feta is lovely and tangy and still safe to eat.

fusilli or other pasta
2 tsp olive oil or rapeseed oil
1 onion
1 clove garlic

2 medium carrots
½ tsp ground cumin
1 x 400g tin chopped tomatoes
1 x 400g tin green or brown lentils (230g drained)
1 tbsp balsamic vinegar
½ tsp dried basil
black pepper
40g feta cheese

Preparation time: 10 minutes plus 10–15 minutes simmering.
Equipment: 1 frying pan with a lid and 1 pan for pasta.
Storage: Fridge for 24 hours or freeze (before adding feta).
Servings: 2.

- Cook the pasta according to the instructions on the packet.
- Peel and dice the onion.
- Heat the oil in the frying pan and sauté the onion with the crushed garlic for a few minutes while you prepare the carrots.
- Peel and coarsely grate the carrots and add to the frying pan. Put a lid on the pan and leave to sweat for a few minutes while you get the other ingredients and drain the lentils.
- Stir the cumin into the pan, then add the tomatoes, lentils, vinegar and basil. Bring to the boil and leave to simmer for about 10 minutes. Add black pepper to taste.
- Drain the pasta and stir in the lentil sauce. Serve and crumble the feta over the top.

Tip

- To reduce your salt and saturated fat intake, you can use a reduced fat version of feta, usually labelled as 'Greek-style cheese' or 'Greek salad cheese' because it's not allowed to be called feta.

Why you should eat a low GI diet

GI stands for glycaemic index, and a low GI diet just means having foods that are broken down slowly, like lentils and oats. Foods that are more refined, such as white bread and sugar, have a high GI. They are digested quickly and result in a rapid increase in blood sugar levels. Low GI foods are digested more slowly, so they lead to much smaller and slower increases and decreases in blood sugar, and keep you feeling full for longer. Low GI regimes designed for weight loss aren't appropriate for pregnancy, but switching to low GI foods will mean you're less likely to put on too much weight while you're pregnant. It will also reduce the risk of having a baby with a neural tube defect, particularly if you're overweight. So instead of choosing white rice, pasta or bread, opt for wholegrain varieties along with lentils, pulses and oats.

Quick vegetable noodles

These are very quick to cook and can be eaten on their own or with a piece of fish or grilled chicken.

½ red pepper
4 broccoli florets (about 150g)
4 mushrooms
2 tsp rapeseed oil
2 cloves garlic
1 tbsp grated fresh root ginger
½ red chilli
4 spring onions
2 portions straight to wok noodles (rice or wheat noodles)
50g frozen soya beans or peas
1 tbsp reduced salt soya sauce
2 tbsp rice vinegar or white wine vinegar
2 tbsp fresh coriander

Preparation time: 15 minutes.
Equipment: 1 deep-sided frying pan or wok.
Storage: Fridge for 24 hours.
Servings: 2.

- Remove the stem and seeds from the pepper and slice thinly. Slice the mushrooms and chop the broccoli florets lengthways into thin pieces.
- Heat the oil in the frying pan and stir-fry the pepper, broccoli and mushrooms over a high heat for about 3–5 minutes along with the crushed garlic, grated ginger and finely chopped chilli.
- Meanwhile thinly slice the spring onions.
- Reduce the heat slightly and add the spring onions, noodles, soya beans, soya sauce, vinegar and coriander leaves. Stir well and continue cooking until everything is cooked through.

Chinese-style sticky aubergine

This is a classic Chinese-style dish of stir-fried aubergine in a richly flavoured sauce. It makes a good side dish for steamed fish or stir-fried chicken, or simply mix it with noodles and have it as it is.

1 tbsp rapeseed oil
1 aubergine
2 cloves garlic
1 tbsp grated fresh root ginger
2 tsp reduced salt soya sauce
3 tbsp rice vinegar
150ml water
3 tbsp hoisin sauce
1 tbsp sesame seeds

Preparation time: 25 minutes.
Equipment: 1 frying pan.
Storage: Fridge for 24 hours or freeze.
Servings: 2.

- Chop the stalk off the aubergine and cut lengthways into 1cm thick slices. Slice these into strips like long chips and cut them into shorter, finger-length chips.
- Heat the oil in the pan and fry the aubergine along with the garlic and ginger for about 5 minutes, until softened and browned.
- Add the soya sauce, vinegar, water and hoisin sauce and simmer for about 15 minutes, until the aubergine is well cooked and the sauce has reduced.
- Sprinkle with sesame seeds and serve.

Avocado and artichoke salad

Artichoke hearts are low in calories and fat but rich in antioxidants and fibre. They're eaten here with avocado for healthy fats, along with watercress and lime juice for a bit of a kick.

1 small avocado
½ tin artichoke hearts or 120g from a jar
5cm cucumber
2 handfuls watercress or baby spinach or lettuce
½ small red onion

1 tsp olive oil
1 tbsp lime juice
¼ tsp white sugar

Preparation time: 10 minutes.
Equipment: 1 bowl.
Storage: Fridge for 24 hours.
Servings: 2–3.

- Cut the avocado into quarters, discard the stone and peel, then slice.
- Cut the artichoke hearts into quarters, slice the cucumber as thinly as possible and remove any thick stems from the watercress.
- Peel and very finely dice the red onion.
- In a small bowl combine the oil, lime juice and sugar to make a dressing.
- Mix the vegetables together and dress the salad.

Tuna niçoise salad

This is a simple but classic dish. When it's made well, the flavours all come together to make something really special. This version contains tinned tuna, boiled eggs, new potatoes and fine green beans in a light dressing to provide a whole range of nutrients that you and your baby need.

300g baby new potatoes
100g fine green beans
2 eggs
1 x 125g tin tuna
2 tsp olive oil or oil from the tin of tuna
2 tsp white wine vinegar
2 tsp lemon juice
2 spring onions
½ tsp wholegrain mustard
1 tomato
handful pitted black olives

Preparation time: 30 minutes.
Equipment: 2 pans and 1 large bowl.
Storage: Fridge for 24 hours or freeze.
Servings: 2.

- Place the new potatoes in a pan, cover with boiling water, bring to the boil and simmer for 20 minutes. Then add the green beans and simmer for 5 minutes more, until the potatoes and beans are both tender.
- Meanwhile, put the eggs in a pan, cover with water, bring to the boil and simmer for 10 minutes. Then drain and refill the pan with cold water.
- Slice the spring onion very thinly. Drain the tuna and place in a bowl with the spring onion, oil, vinegar, lemon juice and mustard and mix well.
- Chop the tomatoes into bite-sized chunks and cut the olives in half. Add to the tuna mixture.
- When the potatoes and beans are ready, drain them and add the beans to the salad bowl. Cut the potatoes into quarters, or just in half if they are very small, and combine gently with the other ingredients. If you want to, you can run cold water over the hot vegetables, but they will cool quickly with the cold salad ingredients and the overall dish tastes nicer slightly warm rather than completely cold.
- If the eggs are too hot to handle, run them under a cold tap for a few seconds. Remove the shell, cut the eggs into quarters and arrange them on top of the salad.

Tips

- Ideally this is made with leftover potatoes and beans from the night before to save on work. If you're using leftovers from the fridge, pop them in the microwave for a minute and this will make the whole dish much more flavourful.
- Instead of green beans you can use tinned white beans, such as butter beans or cannellini beans.

Sea bass with soya and ginger

This is a light, fragrant dish which is very easy to make. It goes perfectly with quick vegetable noodles (p33) or some plain basmati rice and a few vegetables.

2 whole sea bass (cleaned and gutted)
2 carrots
4 spring onions
½–1 red chilli
2–3cm fresh root ginger
1 clove garlic
2 tsp reduced salt soya sauce
1 tsp sesame oil
4 tbsp rice vinegar or white wine vinegar

Preparation time: 10 minutes plus 25 minutes baking.
Equipment: 1 baking tray or large roasting tin.
Storage: Fridge for 24 hours.
Servings: 2.

- Preheat the oven to 200°C (180°C fan)/400°F/gas mark 6.
- Peel the carrots and cut into matchstick-sized pieces. Thinly slice the spring onions and chilli.
- Peel the root ginger and cut into thin slices, then do the same with the garlic.
- Place two large pieces of foil on the baking tray and place one fish on each piece. Put half the carrots, spring onions, chilli, ginger and garlic inside the fish and scatter the remainder on top.
- Sprinkle the soya sauce, sesame oil and vinegar over the fish, then bring up the edges of the foil to meet each other and fold over the top and edges to secure each of the two parcels.
- Place in the oven for 25 minutes, until the fish is completely cooked.

Baked fish with couscous

A simple, light meal with a refreshing lemony taste, which is great if you can't face rich sauces or strong flavours.

125g dry couscous
1 courgette
1 lemon
1 tbsp pine nuts
1 tsp dried parsley
250ml stock
2 firm white fish (such as haddock, cod, coley or river cobbler), gutted and cleaned

Preparation time: 10 minutes plus 30 minutes baking.
Pans: 1 shallow casserole dish with a lid or foil for covering.
Storage: Fridge for 24 hours or freeze.
Servings: 2.

- Preheat the oven to 180°C (160°C fan)/350°F/gas mark 4. Place the pine nuts on a piece of foil and toast under the grill for 1 minute.

- Chop the ends off the courgette, then slice into quarters lengthways and thinly slice.
- Place the couscous, courgette and pinenuts and parsley in the casserole dish and mix.
- Lay the fish fillets side by side on top.
- Cut the lemon in half, then cut off two slices and lay one on top of each piece of fish.
- Make up the stock and add the zest and juice of the remaining lemon.
- Pour the stock over the fish and couscous. Cover with a lid or foil and bake for 25–30 minutes, until the fish is cooked through. The cooking time will depend on the thickness of your fish.

Iodine update

'Iodine is important for the production of thyroid hormones. Recent research has shown the re-emergence of mild iodine deficiency in schoolgirls and pregnant women in the UK. Iodine is essential for the development of the baby's brain during pregnancy and early life. Iodine deficiency in a pregnant woman, even if mild, can lead to impaired brain development in the baby and this can have long-term implications, such as a lower IQ in the child. Good dietary sources include fish, shellfish and dairy products. In the UK, milk and dairy products are the main iodine sources, although organic milk has a 40% lower iodine content than conventional milk. Research carried out here in Surrey found that if women follow the general healthy eating advice for pregnancy and have 2–3 portions of dairy produce a day (such as milk, yogurt, cheese) and 1–2 portions of fish a week they should get enough iodine.'

Margaret Rayman, Professor of Nutritional
Medicine, University of Surrey

Thai-style salmon fishcakes

These are flavoured with ginger, lime and coriander and taste great with stir-fried vegetables and rice or noodles. A little sweet chilli sauce goes very well with them too.

> 2 salmon fillets
> 2 spring onions
> ½ lime
> 1 tbsp grated fresh ginger
> 1 tbsp chopped fresh coriander or ½ tsp ground coriander
> ½–1 red chilli (optional)
> 1 egg
> 1 tbsp oats
> 1 tbsp sesame seeds
> 2 tsp rapeseed oil

Preparation time: 15 minutes plus 5 minutes cooking.
Equipment: 1 frying pan and 1 mixing bowl.
Storage: Fridge for 24 hours or freeze.
Servings: 2.

- Chop the salmon into pea-sized pieces. The quickest way to do this is to cut the fillets into long strips, then put these together and slice them.
- Finely chop the spring onions and place in a bowl with the salmon, the zest of ½ a lime and 1 tbsp of lime juice, ginger, coriander, finely chopped chilli (if using), egg, oats and sesame seeds.
- Mix well. You can use the mixture straightaway or cover the bowl and leave it in the fridge for a few hours.
- Heat the oil in a frying pan and when it is sizzling spoon the salmon mixture into four heaps to form the fishcakes.
- Flatten with the back of a spoon and cook for 2–3 minutes. Carefully turn over, then cook the other side.

15-minute pasta with chicken and broccoli

A really quick and simple recipe made with very few ingredients but packed with antioxidants and other essential nutrients.

> fusilli or other pasta
> 2 tsp olive oil or rapeseed oil
> 250g diced chicken
> 1 clove garlic
> 200g broccoli

1 tbsp wholegrain mustard
3 tbsp orange juice
2 tbsp pine nuts or flaked almonds

Preparation time: 15 minutes.
Equipment: 1 pan for pasta, 1 small bowl and 1 deep-sided frying pan.
Storage: Fridge for 24 hours or freeze.
Servings: 2.

- Cook the pasta according to the instructions on the packet.
- Chop the chicken into bite-sized chunks if not already cut.
- Heat the oil in the frying pan and fry the chicken for 2–3 minutes, until starting to brown.
- Meanwhile chop the broccoli into bite-sized pieces.
- Add the crushed garlic to the chicken and stir, then mix in the broccoli and cook for another 5 minutes.
- Meanwhile, place the pine nuts on a piece of foil and toast under the grill for 1–2 minutes.
- In a small bowl, combine the mustard and orange juice. Stir this into the chicken and broccoli, along with 3 tablespoons of the pasta water, and leave to cook for 2 minutes.
- Drain the pasta and combine with the other ingredients.
- Divide between two bowls and sprinkle with pine nuts.

Sesame chicken

This is incredibly easy to make and tastes as good as, if not better than, in any Chinese restaurant. Perfect with stir-fried vegetables and basmati rice.

2 chicken breasts
1 egg
1 heaped tbsp plain flour
1 heaped tbsp cornflour
2 tsp rapeseed oil

Sauce
1 tbsp honey
2 tsp reduced salt soya sauce
1 tsp sesame oil
1 tbsp tomato puree

1 tbsp rice wine vinegar or white wine vinegar
1 clove garlic, crushed
1 tsp grated fresh root ginger
1 tbsp sesame seeds
½ tsp cornflour

To serve
1 tsp sesame seeds

Preparation time: 25 minutes.
Equipment: 1 mixing bowl and 1 frying pan.
Storage: Fridge for 24 hours or freeze.
Servings: 2.

- Crack the egg into the bowl and, using a fork, beat lightly with the flour and cornflour.
- Cut the chicken into bite-sized pieces and stir into the egg mixture.
- In a small bowl or cup, mix together all the ingredients for the sauce.
- Heat the oil in the frying pan and when it's really hot, tip in the chicken mixture. Fry over a medium to high heat for about 5 minutes, using a fish slice or spatula to turn over the chicken and separate the pieces.
- When the chicken is nicely browned all over, turn the heat down to medium and pour the sauce over the chicken. Stir and fry for another 5 minutes, until the chicken is well cooked through, then turn off the heat and sprinkle with the remaining sesame seeds.

Why you should cook chicken carefully

Chicken is very versatile and nutritious: high in protein, niacin and selenium and low in saturated fat, provided you remove the skin and don't cook it in lots of fat. However, while you're pregnant, you do need to be especially careful when you're cooking chicken to avoid a dose of salmonella. As well as making sure it's thoroughly cooked, you should keep raw chicken away from other foods and wash your hands and any cooking equipment to prevent cross-contamination. It's not a good idea to wash raw chicken, as splashes of water can spread salmonella. It's also best to have a chopping board that is only ever used for *raw* meat, poultry and fish.

Vinegar and tarragon braised chicken

A satisfying dish with a gentle but definite vinegary flavour. It's made with chicken thighs rather than breast portions for extra iron. It was specially created for those craving vinegary flavours but trying not to overdo the salt and vinegar crisps and pickles – you can even sprinkle a little more vinegar on at the end if you like.

4 chicken thigh fillets (skinless and boneless)
freshly ground black pepper
2 tsp rapeseed oil
2 cloves garlic
6 shallots
75ml white wine vinegar
1 tbsp honey
100ml stock
½ tsp Dijon mustard
1 tbsp chopped fresh tarragon or 1 tsp dried tarragon
1 tbsp chopped fresh parsley or 1 tsp dried parsley
extra parsley for garnish (optional)

Preparation time: 15 minutes plus 15 minutes simmering.
Equipment: 1 frying pan with a lid.
Storage: Fridge for 24 hours or freeze.
Servings: 2–3.

- Grind some black pepper over the chicken thighs.
- Heat the oil in the pan over a high heat and sear the chicken for about 5 minutes, turning so that all sides begin to brown slightly. When done, move the chicken from the pan to a plate.
- Meanwhile, peel and dice the shallots.
- Turn the heat down slightly and sauté the shallots with the crushed garlic for about 3 minutes, until softened.
- Add the vinegar and honey and simmer for about 5 minutes, until the liquid has reduced by about half.
- Add the mustard, herbs and stock and bring back to the boil, then return the chicken and simmer with the lid on for 15 minutes, until the chicken is cooked through. Turn the chicken over halfway through to ensure even cooking.
- Serve sprinkled with extra parsley.

Sausage and bean casserole

This recipe combines Quorn sausages or good-quality lean pork sausages with plenty of veg and a rich tomato sauce for a healthy supper. Great with baked or mashed potato but also good with pasta or rice too.

4 sausages (Quorn or lean pork)
1 small onion
1 clove garlic
½ red pepper
2 tsp olive oil or rapeseed oil
1 x 210g tin kidney beans
1 x 400g tin chopped tomatoes
1 tbsp tomato puree
1 bay leaf
1 tsp mixed herbs
¼ tsp smoked paprika or regular paprika
¼ tsp sugar
salt and pepper

Preparation time: 10 minutes plus 20 minutes or longer simmering time.
Equipment: 1 casserole pan with a lid.
Storage: Fridge for 24 hours or freeze.
Servings: 2.

- Cook the sausages in the oven or under the grill according to the instructions.
- Peel and dice the onion. Remove the stalk and seeds from the pepper, then dice.
- Heat the oil in the pan and sauté the onion, pepper and crushed garlic for 5 minutes.
- Add the chopped tomatoes, kidney beans, tomato puree, bay leaf, herbs, paprika, sugar, a pinch of salt and some black pepper. Bring to the boil, then leave to simmer for at least 15 minutes.
- As soon as the sausages are cooked, add them to the pan and cover with the sauce. Cook in the sauce for at least 5 minutes. Cooking for longer (maybe 15 minutes) is better and will help all the flavours come together.

Moussaka

A healthier version of the traditional Greek dish that you can make with Quorn mince or minced lamb. It's packed with vegetables and tastes good with rice or crusty bread and maybe a little side salad.

1 aubergine
2 tsp olive oil or rapeseed oil
1 small onion
2 cloves garlic
1 small courgette
½ tsp cinnamon
½ tsp dried mixed herbs
½ tsp dried parsley
4 mint leaves or ¼ tsp dried mint
1 bay leaf
150g Quorn mince or lean minced lamb
1 x 400g tin chopped tomatoes
1 tbsp tomato puree
salt and freshly ground black pepper

Topping
200ml milk
10g butter or margarine
2 level tbsp plain flour
1 bay leaf
pinch ground nutmeg
1 heaped tbsp pecorino or Parmesan cheese

Preparation time: 40 minutes plus 20–25 minutes baking.
Equipment: 1 baking tray, 1 deep-sided frying pan, 1 small saucepan and 1 ovenproof dish.
Storage: Fridge for 24 hours or freeze.
Servings: 2–3.

- Preheat the oven to 230°C (210°C fan)/450°F/gas mark 8.
- Cut the aubergine into 1cm thick slices. Use 1 teaspoon of the oil to brush over both sides of the slices, then arrange them in a single layer on the baking tray and bake for about 20 minutes, until browned. Don't worry if the slices seem slightly dry as they are going to cook further in the sauce.

- Meanwhile, peel and dice the onion. Heat the remaining oil in the frying pan and sauté the onion and crushed garlic for 2–3 minutes.
- Coarsely grate the courgette, add to the pan and cook for 3 minutes more, until softened.
- If you are using lamb you should now turn up the heat, add the lamb and cook for a few minutes to brown. If you're using Quorn you can add it after the spices.
- Add the cinnamon, mixed herbs, parsley, bay leaf and chopped mint leaves to the pan and stir.
- Stir in the tin of tomatoes, tomato puree and Quorn if using. Bring to the boil, then simmer gently while you prepare the rest.
- Place the milk, butter or margarine, flour, bay leaf and nutmeg in a pan. Stir over a medium heat until simmering, then turn down the heat, continue stirring, and simmer for a few more minutes to thicken. Take off the heat.
- Remove the aubergine from the oven and turn down the temperature to 200°C (180°C fan)/400°F/gas mark 6.
- Grate the pecorino cheese.
- Spoon half the mince mixture into the ovenproof dish, then layer half the aubergine on top. Repeat the layers, then pour the white sauce over the top and sprinkle on the cheese.
- Place in the oven for 20–25 minutes, until bubbling at the edges and nicely browned.

Hearty beef stew

If comfort food is what you're looking for just now, this is perfect. A traditional beef stew, without the wine but with tender beef, potatoes and vegetables in a rich, tasty sauce.

1 tbsp rapeseed oil or olive oil
1 onion
1 leek
600g lean beef or stewing steak
2 tbsp plain flour
salt and pepper
4 carrots
4 parsnips
2–3 medium potatoes (about 500g unpeeled)
2 tbsp tomato puree
2 tbsp Worcestershire sauce

> 2 bay leaves
> 1 tbsp chopped fresh herbs (thyme and rosemary) or 1 tsp dried mixed herbs
> 550ml beef or vegetable stock

Preparation time: 30 minutes plus 3 hours cooking.
Equipment: 1 ovenproof saucepan or casserole dish with a lid.
Storage: Fridge for 24 hours or freeze.
Servings: 4.

- Preheat the oven to 180°C (160°C fan)/350°F/gas mark 4.
- Cut the beef into 2cm pieces if not already cut. Put the flour on a plate with a little salt and pepper and toss the beef to coat it.
- Peel and dice the onion. Wash the leek, then top and tail it and slice in half lengthways. Wash again if needed, then finely slice.
- Heat the oil in the pan and fry the onion and leek for about 5 minutes, until translucent.
- Meanwhile, peel and chop the potatoes, carrots and parsnips into 1–2cm pieces.
- Add the beef, vegetables and other ingredients to the pan and gently stir. Bring to the boil with the lid on, then place in the oven for 3 hours. Remove the lid for the last half hour to reduce and thicken the sauce.

Tips

- Other vegetables that go very well in the stew are butternut squash, sweet potato, turnips and mushrooms.
- You can replace half the stock with red wine if you prefer (see p135).

Desserts and snacks

Blueberry compote with lemon yogurt

This delicious compote is rich in antioxidants and tastes great with tangy lemon yogurt. It also goes well with plain yogurt or on top of pancakes or porridge.

> *Blueberry compote*
> 350g frozen blueberries
> 1 star anise
> 1 stick of cinnamon or ½ tsp ground cinnamon

juice of ½ a lemon
1 tbsp honey

Lemon yogurt
400g low fat natural yogurt
1 tbsp runny honey
zest of ½ a lemon

Preparation time: 5 minutes plus 15 minutes simmering.
Equipment: 1 pan.
Storage: Fridge for 24 hours or freeze.
Servings: 4.

- Put about half the blueberries into the pan with the star anise, cinnamon, lemon juice and honey.
- Heat until nearly boiling and simmer for 10 minutes.
- Stir well so that the blueberries start to mash, then add the remaining blueberries, turn up the heat and simmer for 2–3 minutes more.
- Allow to cool while combining the lemony yogurt ingredients. Serve together.

Poached pink pears

Poached pears always look quite decadent and the colour of these makes them look extra special. However, they're very healthy and perfect for breakfast with some natural yogurt or served with cream or ice cream at a dinner party.

4 pears
4 plums
250g frozen mixed berries
50g dried apricots
100ml orange juice or red grape juice
1 tsp cinnamon
2 tsp soft brown sugar

Preparation time: 10 minutes plus 15–25 minutes simmering.
Equipment: 1 pan.
Storage: Fridge for 24 hours or freeze.
Servings: 4–5 portions.

- Cut the pears into quarters and remove the peel and core.
- Chop the plums in half and remove the stones but leave the skin on.
- Put the pears into the pan, then add the apricots, plums, berries, sugar, cinnamon and orange juice. Bring to the boil, then simmer for about 15–25 minutes, depending on the ripeness and size of the pears and plums, until the fruit is soft.
- Serve warm or cold.

Osborne pudding

Osborne pudding is a traditional English dish made with brown bread and marmalade. It's said to have been a favourite of Queen Victoria, and while this is made with less sugar and fat than the one she would have eaten, it still tastes like old-school comfort food. It goes well with custard, vanilla ice cream or reduced fat crème fraîche.

4 slices of wholemeal bread
25g butter, margarine or reduced fat spread
60g marmalade
60g dried apricots
zest of ½ an orange
pinch of nutmeg
350ml milk
2 eggs
1 tsp soft brown sugar
1 tsp vanilla essence

Preparation time: 15 minutes plus 20 minutes baking.
Equipment: 1 ovenproof dish, 1 pan and 1 bowl.
Storage: Fridge for 24 hours or freeze.
Servings: 4–6.

- Preheat the oven to 180°C (160°C fan)/350°F/gas mark 4.
- Grease the ovenproof dish with a little of the butter, then spread the rest on the bread, followed by the marmalade.
- Coarsely chop the apricots.
- Cut each slice of bread diagonally into four triangles. Place half the pieces in a layer on the bottom of the dish, then scatter the apricots on top followed by the rest of the bread.
- Grate the orange zest on top and sprinkle on the nutmeg.

- Put the milk in a pan or microwaveable jug and heat until steaming hot but not quite boiling.
- Meanwhile, crack the eggs into a bowl and beat with the sugar and vanilla essence.
- When the milk is hot, slowly pour it into the egg mixture as you stir.
- Pour the mixture over the bread and leave to soak for 5 minutes. If any corners of bread are sticking up, you can press them down with the back of a spoon.
- Place in the oven for 20 minutes, until nicely browned on top.

Triple ginger cookies

These are made with three different types of ginger to give them a perfect flavour and extra power for fighting off morning sickness.

75ml rapeseed oil
1 egg
175g self-raising flour
1 tsp bicarbonate of soda
100g soft brown sugar
2½ tsp ground ginger
1 heaped tbsp grated fresh root ginger
75g crystallised ginger
1 tbsp golden syrup

Preparation time: 15 minutes plus 10 minutes baking.
Equipment: 1 mixing bowl and 2 baking trays.
Storage: Airtight container for a few days or freeze.
Servings: 16–18 cookies.

- Preheat the oven to 180°C (160°C fan)/350°F/gas mark 4.
- Measure the oil into a jug and use a little of it to brush over the baking trays.
- Crack the egg into the remaining oil in the jug and beat lightly with a fork.
- Place the flour, bicarbonate of soda, brown sugar and ground ginger in the mixing bowl.
- Finely chop the crystallised ginger. Add it and the grated fresh ginger to the bowl.
- Add the egg mixture and the syrup to the bowl and mix.
- Using your hands, bring all the ingredients together to form a ball.

- Take a walnut-sized piece of the dough, roll it into a ball and flatten gently between your hands so that it is about 0.5cm thick. Make 16–18 cookies like this and place them on the trays.
- Bake for 10 minutes, until golden brown.
- Leave the cookies to cool and set on the trays for 5 minutes, then use a fish slice or spatula to move them to a cooling rack.

Fact or fiction: Ginger is a good cure for morning sickness

It certainly is. In fact there is stronger scientific support for eating ginger than for any other morning sickness remedy (excluding drug treatments for women with extremely severe sickness). If you're suffering from waves of nausea or spending most of the day feeling not quite right, then give ginger a try. Trials show that the majority of women having ginger feel less nauseous and vomit less often. These triple ginger cookies contain much more ginger than ginger snap biscuits you might buy, which probably won't contain enough to have an effect. You may need to have ginger three or four times a day to reap the benefits and you can do this by also having ginger tea and grated ginger in soups and stir-fries, or by buying ginger sweets or chews.

Chocolate and ginger refrigerator slices

These rich chocolaty treats don't need any cooking and are ideal if you're not feeling great and fancy something sweet. You can adjust the ginger to make them more spicy or less, according to taste.

100g stem ginger
75g dried apricots
75g raisins
200g stem ginger cookies or gingernut biscuits
200g dark chocolate
100g milk chocolate
75g golden syrup
100g butter or soya margarine

Preparation time: 25 minutes plus 2 hours in the fridge.
Equipment: 1 large bowl and 1 baking tray (20cm x 30cm).
Storage: Fridge for 3–4 days or freeze.
Servings: 32 slices.

- Put the kettle on or start heating a pan of water.
- Cover a baking tray with a piece of greaseproof paper.
- Finely chop the ginger and apricots on a chopping board. Chop the biscuits roughly into 1cm pieces.
- Heat a large bowl over a pan of just simmering water. Break the chocolate into the bowl and add the syrup and butter or margarine. Stir until the chocolate has melted and you have a smooth mixture.
- Take the bowl off the heat and stir in the biscuits, ginger, apricots and raisins.
- Pour the mixture into the prepared tray and smooth down lightly with the back of a spoon so it fills the whole tray. Leave to cool for 10 minutes, then cover with cling film and place in the fridge for 2 hours, until set.
- Cut into 32 slices by first cutting it into 4 strips lengthways, then cutting each strip into 8 pieces.

Tips

- If you want to make these more gingery, add an additional 25g of stem ginger. For a less gingery version, replace 50g of ginger with dried fruit.
- Try other dried fruits such as cranberries or dates, or add some flaked almonds or chopped hazelnuts.

Oat and raisin cookies

Ideal if you're feeling extra hungry or just want something sweet. They're made with oats and juicy raisins for extra nutrients.

1 egg
125ml rapeseed oil, plus extra for greasing
2 tbsp milk
75g dark muscovado sugar
100g oats
50g wholemeal flour
50g plain flour
½ tsp baking powder
½ tsp bicarbonate of soda
75g raisins

Preparation time: 15 minutes plus 10 minutes baking.
Equipment: 1 mixing bowl and 2 baking trays.
Storage: Airtight container for a few days or freeze.
Servings: 16 cookies.

- Preheat the oven to 200°C (180°C fan)/400°F/gas mark 6. Grease two baking trays.
- Measure the oil in a jug or bowl, then crack the egg into it, add the milk and beat lightly.
- Put the sugar into the mixing bowl and break up any lumps with the back of a spoon. Add the oats, flour, baking powder and bicarbonate of soda.
- Stir, then make a well in the centre and pour in the oil mixture. Mix, then fold in the raisins.
- Place dessertspoonfuls of the mixture onto the trays. Spread the mixture out with the back of a spoon to make cookies and place them in the oven for 10 minutes, until nicely browned.
- Leave to cool on the trays for 5–10 minutes before transferring to a cooling rack.

Tip

- You can spice these up by adding 1–2 teaspoons of mixed spice or ground ginger.

Why you should cook with rapeseed oil

Rapeseed oil, known as canola oil in the United States, contains a healthier balance of fatty acids than either butter or margarine. It contains just 6% saturated fat, compared with 52% in butter, 10% in sunflower margarine or oil and 14% in olive oil. Instead, rapeseed oil contains more of the beneficial monounsaturated and polyunsaturated fats, so it's better for your blood cholesterol levels and your heart. It doesn't have a very strong flavour, which makes it ideal for baking, when you want the taste of the other ingredients such as fruit, vanilla or chocolate to shine through. Other oils, such as olive and sesame oil, can add to the flavour of dishes like pasta or stir-fries, and rapeseed oil has a higher smoking point, which means it's more stable at high temperatures, making it good for frying.

Marmalade flapjacks

These make a nice, tangy treat, with treacle and dried apricots for extra iron and oats for slow-release energy.

300g oats
50g walnuts (optional)
150g dried apricots

125g thick-cut marmalade
2 tbsp treacle
125ml rapeseed oil

Preparation time: 15 minutes plus 20 minutes baking.
Equipment: 1 pan and 1 baking tray (25cm x 25cm).
Storage: Airtight container for a few days or freeze.
Servings: 16 flapjacks.

- Preheat the oven to 180°C (160°C fan)/350°F/gas mark 4.
- Line the baking tray with greaseproof paper.
- Place the marmalade, treacle and oil in a large pan, heat gently and stir until the ingredients are combined. Then turn off the heat and leave to cool for a few minutes.
- Chop the apricots and walnuts (if using).
- Add the oats, walnuts and apricots to the pan and stir well.
- Turn out the mixture onto the baking tray and smooth out as evenly as possible. Bake for 20 minutes, until the edges look cooked but the centre is still soft.
- Leave to cool on the baking tray for 5 minutes, then mark with three lines across and three lines downwards to make 16 flapjacks. Remove and leave to cool on a cooling rack.

Crunchy chickpea mix

Perfect with a mocktail and a lovely substitute for crisps or roasted peanuts, with less fat but more flavour.

1 x 400g tin chickpeas
2 tsp rapeseed oil
½ tsp paprika
¼ tsp mild chilli powder (more if you like)
½ tsp ground cumin
½ tsp ground coriander
½ tsp mixed herbs
pinch of salt
black pepper
25g Brazil nuts or other nuts (whole or roughly cut)
25g pumpkin seeds

Preparation time: 5 minutes plus 1 hour baking.
Equipment: 1 bowl and 1 baking tray.
Storage: Airtight container for 2–3 days.
Servings: 3–4.

- Preheat the oven to 160°C (140°C fan)/325°F/gas mark 3.
- Drain the chickpeas and tip into the bowl. Add all the other ingredients, apart from the nuts and seeds.
- Mix well, then transfer to the baking tray and place in the oven for 50 minutes. Keep the bowl and put the nuts and seeds into it. Stir to coat them with any remaining oil and spices.
- After 50 minutes, mix the nuts and seeds with the chickpeas and bake for another 10 minutes.
- Leave to cool before transferring to an airtight container.

Drinks

Ginger tea

This is very simple to make and you can drink it as it is, sweeten it, or add some lemon for extra flavour. You can also choose whether to drink it warm or put it in the fridge and have it cold.

2–3cm fresh root ginger
1 mug of boiling water
1–2 tsp honey or sugar (optional)
1 tsp (a squeeze) lemon or lime juice (optional)

Preparation time: 2 minutes plus 10–15 minutes steeping.
Equipment: 1 mug.
Storage: Drink straightaway or fridge for 24 hours.
Servings: 1.

- Peel the ginger, then either grate it into your mug, slice it or cut it into chunks.
- Pour over boiling water and leave for 10–15 minutes.
- Taste it, then, if you want to, add some honey or lemon.

Tips

- Some people also like to add a mint leaf to the ginger before pouring in the boiling water.

- You can strain it if you want to or just leave the bits of ginger in and throw them away once you've drunk the tea.
- Although ginger is considered safe for pregnancy, some experts believe you shouldn't drink more than 3–4 cups a day, as a precaution.

Mocktails

Why you should swap cocktails for mocktails

Everyone knows that big boozy nights out aren't a good idea when you're pregnant. But what about the odd drink on a special occasion or a glass of wine with dinner at the weekend? The bottom line is that nobody knows how much alcohol you could drink without it affecting your baby. There is no evidence that a couple of units of alcohol once or twice a week causes any harm, but experts can't be 100% sure. So the current advice is not to drink any alcohol at all while you're pregnant. Drinking is associated with an increased risk of miscarriage in early pregnancy. Drinking more than about 10 units a week increases the risks of your baby having limb and heart defects and developmental problems. Recent research suggests genetics also play a role and babies with certain genes are better able to break down alcohol than others.

Apple and ginger fizz

A refreshing drink and especially good for nausea – but be sure to look for ginger ale that says on the label it's made with 'real ginger' or check the ingredients list for 'ginger extract'.

100ml pure apple juice (pressed juice if possible)
200ml ginger ale
¼ fresh lime

- Fill a tall glass with ice.
- Pour in the apple juice and ginger ale.
- Squeeze in the juice of the lime and stir.

Orange and cranberry sunrise

This looks like a real cocktail so you don't feel you're missing out.

75ml orange juice
75ml cranberry juice
75ml sparkling water or soda water

- To get a layered sunrise effect, pour in the orange juice first, add plenty of ice then slowly pour in the cranberry juice and water.

Sunshine sangria

A non-alcoholic version of the traditional holiday drink. Great for barbecues or summer evenings.

1 orange
1 apple
1 lemon
350ml red grape juice
250ml orange juice
250ml sparkling water

Preparation time: 10 minutes plus 1 hour in the fridge if possible.
Equipment: 1 jug.
Storage: Fridge for 1–2 days
Servings: 4–6.

- Wash the fruit. Cut the ends off the orange then cut in half and slice into half rounds.
- Quarter the apple, remove the core then slice thinly. Place the orange and apple slices in the jug and squeeze over the lemon juice.
- Add the grape juice and orange juice then cover with cling film and leave in the fridge for an hour while the flavours develop.
- When ready to serve, add the sparkling water and serve in wine glasses with a few ice cubes.

Tip

- You can also add some fresh mint leaves and sliced strawberries.

Almost mulled wine

Perfect for chilly evenings, especially bonfire night or Christmas and New Year's get-togethers.

1 clementine
2 cloves
1 star anise
1 cinnamon stick
pinch freshly ground nutmeg
2 tsp honey
300ml red grape juice
200ml apple juice
100ml water

Preparation time: 5 minutes plus 15 minutes simmering.
Equipment: 1 pan.
Storage: Drink straightaway.
Servings: 2–3.

- Cut the clementine, including the skin, into quarters and place in the pan along with all the other ingredients.
- Stir and bring almost to the boil, then reduce the heat and simmer for about 15 minutes.

Fact or fiction: Fruit juice is as bad for you as cola

Fruit juice has received a lot of bad press recently and it's easy to drink too much of it, but there's no question that it's better for you than a can of cola. Fizzy drinks such as cola and lemonade contain empty calories, which means they provide energy but not the vitamins and minerals your baby needs. Fruit juices contain sugars too, but they also provide vitamins, minerals and beneficial phytochemicals, especially antioxidants, which are important for your baby's developing immune system. So, while drinking a few glasses of fruit juice every day isn't advisable, especially if you're overweight, most mums-to-be can enjoy a few glasses a week, safe in the knowledge that it's a healthy choice.

First trimester meal planner

You don't need to follow a meal plan while you're pregnant, and if you're suffering from morning sickness it may be completely unrealistic to try at this stage. However, the plan laid out here shows what a healthy diet looks like for the first trimester. It includes plenty of fruit and vegetables, some starchy carbohydrate-rich foods with each meal, and a few snack foods too.

This meal plan meets the requirements for energy, protein, potassium, calcium, magnesium, phosphorus, iron, copper, zinc, chloride, selenium, iodine, thiamin, riboflavin, niacin and vitamins A, B6, B12, C and E.

To meet all the nutrient requirements for this stage of pregnancy, you would also need to take a supplement containing 400µg folic acid and 10µg vitamin D (see p9) and have plenty of water or other drinks.

Day 1

Breakfast: Cinnamon and banana porridge (p17)
Lunch: Creamy butternut squash and red pepper soup (p22), a granary roll, a slice of Cheddar, 2 satsumas
Dinner: 15-minute pasta with chicken and broccoli (p39), poached pink pears (p47) with reduced fat crème fraîche
Snacks: Triple ginger cookie (p49), decaf cappuccino, an apple

Day 2

Breakfast: Glass of orange juice, branflakes with semi-skimmed milk
Lunch: 2 thick slices of wholemeal toast with smoked mackerel pâté (p27) and sliced tomato
Dinner: Sausage and bean casserole (p43) with mashed potato and cabbage, a fruit yogurt
Snacks: Houmous with carrot and breadsticks, a pear

Day 3

Breakfast: 2 slices of thick wholemeal toast with peanut butter, a fruit yogurt

Lunch: Courgette, ricotta and basil frittata (p25), green salad with vinaigrette, a granary roll with spread
Dinner: Hearty beef stew (p45), banana with yogurt, honey and flaked almonds
Snacks: Triple ginger cookie (p49)

Day 4

Breakfast: Made-to-measure muesli (p19) with milk and strawberries
Lunch: Baked potato with baked beans and reduced fat Cheddar, an orange
Dinner: Thai-style salmon fishcakes (p38) with quick vegetable noodles (p33)
Snacks: Rice cakes with reduced fat cream cheese, dried apricots, a chocolate digestive

Day 5

Breakfast: Branflakes with milk and sliced banana
Lunch: Chicken salad wrap, packet of crisps, an apple
Dinner: Vegetarian pizza, avocado and artichoke salad (p34)
Snacks: Apple and ginger fizz (p55), mixed fruit and nuts

Day 6

Breakfast: Granary toast with scrambled eggs and grilled tomatoes
Lunch: Rye bread with Gruyère cheese, an apple
Dinner. Fusilli with lentils and feta (p31)
Snacks: Banana bread (p20), oatcakes

Day 7

Breakfast: Banana bread (p20), orange juice
Lunch: Chicken noodle soup (p23)
Dinner: Aubergine and bean burgers (p29), easy sweet potato wedges (p81), ketchup, corn on the cob
Snacks: A peach, small pot of natural yogurt, mixed nuts

3 The second trimester

The second trimester of pregnancy is often more enjoyable than the first. You've had time to get used to the idea of having a baby, morning sickness should be passing and hopefully you'll be feeling less tired and more energised.

If you felt slightly overwhelmed with everything in the first trimester and healthy eating wasn't uppermost in your mind, now is the time for a new start. You have as much as six months left in which to provide your baby with good nutrition. What you eat between now and the birth will have a big effect on her health. It may help to look back at the guidelines (p3) to see where you need to make changes, then try to establish some good eating habits, with three meals a day and some healthy snacks.

This section of the book contains a real mixture of recipes to make it easy for you to get all the nutrients you need. There are hot and cold breakfast ideas and suggestions for wraps and salads that make good lunches. Taking the time to have a healthy meal in the middle of the day can help avoid energy slumps in the afternoon as well as providing extra nutrients. There are several fish recipes – if you've never been a fan, now is a good time to experiment with different types and alternative ways of cooking them. Fish is enormously beneficial during pregnancy (pp90 and 129) and increasing your intake is something really positive you can do for your baby and yourself. Have a look through the other sections of the book, too, for other fish recipes to try.

If you've been suffering from morning sickness, this will most likely start to ease. If you still have periods of nausea, however, make sure you rest as much as possible and use the ginger recipes in Chapter 2 to help relieve the symptoms. As you feel better you may find your appetite returns with gusto, but avoid unhealthy snacks if possible. Instead, try to stick to fruit, yogurt, cereal and other healthy snacks, at least most of the time (p15)!

Feeling deprived

At this stage of pregnancy you may be feeling more like your old self, but slightly disconcerted to see the wine- and Brie-free days stretching out before you. If there's something on the banned list you're beginning to obsess about, do try to think of an alternative. There really is very little that's completely banned during pregnancy – have a look back at the table on p7 and you may find inspiration for safe alternatives. If it's indulgent puddings you're missing, there are pregnancy-friendly recipes for chocolate mousse and tiramisu at the end of this chapter, which you can enjoy without having to worry about raw eggs or other dangers.

During this second trimester your bump will expand nicely and you'll start to feel your baby moving around. As well as a growing waistline, you may also notice your hips and thighs expanding and probably other parts of your body too. Some women notice their back or their arms become wobblier. This is a normal part of pregnancy as your body lays down fat stores to be used in late pregnancy, when your baby will be growing rapidly, and for breastfeeding. However, keep an eye on your weight and don't be tempted to use pregnancy as an excuse for overindulging. If you haven't weighed yourself recently, it's a good idea to do so now. You may have read that women don't need to gain any weight in the first trimester of pregnancy, but in reality most do put on a few pounds. If you have already gained more than that, it's not too late to take control and aim for a more sensible weight gain from now on. While you shouldn't diet to lose weight while you're pregnant, research has shown that women who make conscious or, even better, written plans to eat a healthy diet are less likely to put on too much weight while they're pregnant.

Watch your weight

During the second and third trimesters of pregnancy you should put on about 1 pound (just under 0.5kg) a week, if you were a healthy weight before you became pregnant. A healthy weight gain if you were overweight before becoming pregnant is about half this amount each week.

If you find you're putting on more weight than you'd like, it can be tempting to think you won't worry about it for now and you'll just lose the extra pounds after you have your baby. However, putting on too much weight increases the risk of problems during pregnancy and many women find it harder than they expect to lose those post-baby pounds. For every celebrity who gets back into her size zero jeans in a couple of weeks, there's a gym full of women still wearing their maternity clothes. It's better to eat sensibly now than to overindulge and then try to diet and exercise while looking after a new baby. It doesn't need to be a chore. There are plenty of healthy foods that taste delicious, and you can still have chocolate or crisps or whatever it is you fancy, just not all the time.

Healthy pregnancy swaps

Instead of . . .	Have . . .
Sausages	Salmon – it contains less saturated fat and more omega 3s for your baby's brain development
Crisps	Plain popcorn or some nuts and seeds – these are more filling and contain protein, healthy fats and a range of vitamins and minerals
Sweets	Dried apricots, figs or raisins – these still taste sweet but provide extra vitamins and iron
Bacon sandwich on white bread	Scrambled egg on wholemeal toast – less saturated fat and more iodine, vitamin E, iron and fibre
Cakes and muffins	Bowl of wholegrain cereal – helps with the mid-afternoon energy slump and keeps you going for longer
Biscuits	Rice cakes with reduced fat cream cheese – more calcium but less fat and sugar
Ice cream	Strawberries or banana with a scoop of frozen yogurt – still a treat but less fat and sugar and more micronutrients
Can of coke	Small fruit smoothie – a range of vitamins and minerals rather than just sugar and calories

When you swap highly refined foods such as biscuits and crisps for foods that are more natural, like nuts and fruit, you increase your intake of vitamins and minerals while generally reducing your calorie intake. This is because unrefined foods are bulkier and take more effort to chew and longer to digest, so both your mind and your body are more likely to feel satisfied and register that you've eaten something. That said, don't go mad and snack on dried fruit and nuts all day. If weight is an issue for you, then an apple or other fresh fruit would be a better option, or some vegetable sticks.

In the third trimester you'll find you naturally slow down a bit as your bump grows bigger, but for now try to stay as active as possible. You might need to change the kind of exercise you do, but there's no need to stop, unless you have particular health problems. Walk whenever you can and take gentle exercise when there's time. You'll reap the benefits, having more energy in the day and sleeping better at night.

Breakfasts

Carrot cake porridge

Instant flavoured oats don't even come close to this delicious breakfast. It's packed with natural flavour and you're starting your day with a portion of fruit and vegetables without even noticing.

> 40g oats
> 1 small apple
> 1 small carrot
> 1 tbsp sultanas or raisins
> ½ tsp ground cinnamon
> 225ml milk or a mixture of milk and water
> 1 tsp honey or brown sugar
> 1 rounded tbsp natural yogurt
> 1 tbsp chopped walnuts

Preparation time: 5 minutes plus 5–7 minutes cooking.
Equipment: 1 pan.
Storage: Eat straightaway.
Servings: 1.

- Peel and finely grate the carrot into the pan. Cut the apple into quarters, peel and core it and finely grate it into the pan.
- Add the oats, sultanas, cinnamon and milk to the pan and stir. Bring to the boil on a high heat, then reduce the heat and leave to bubble gently for a few minutes until thickened.
- Pour into a bowl, drizzle honey on top, dollop a large spoonful of yogurt in the middle, then sprinkle with walnuts.

> 66 *I am addicted to this carrot cake porridge! It makes a really hearty, filling breakfast that is much tastier than my usual porridge and the creaminess from the yogurt and crunch of the walnuts are delicious.* 99
> **Magda, 24 weeks pregnant**

Honey nut granola

Delicious with yogurt and fresh berries or just with milk. This is made with less sugar than shop-bought versions and lots more nutrient-packed nuts, seeds and fruit to give you and your baby a really good start to the day.

250g porridge oats
2 tbsp rapeseed oil
100g honey
25g sesame seeds
30g flaked almonds
30g Brazil nuts
25g pumpkin seeds
20g sunflower seeds
50g dried apricots
50g sultanas

Preparation time: 10 minutes plus 25 minutes baking.
Equipment: 1 large pan and 2 baking trays.
Storage: Airtight container for 2–3 weeks.
Servings: 10–12.

- Preheat the oven to 140°C (120°C fan)/275°F/gas mark 1.
- Chop the Brazil nuts and the apricots.
- Put the oil and honey into the pan, stir and heat until it melts and comes together, then turn off the heat.
- Stir in the oats and sesame seeds followed by the other nuts and seeds.
- Spread the mixture out over two baking trays and bake for 20 minutes. Halfway through give the mixture a stir and swap the trays around.
- Stir the fruit into the oat mixture and bake for another 5 minutes.
- Leave to cool, then transfer to an airtight container.

Tips

- You can adjust this basic recipe to include your favourite nuts, seeds and dried fruit. You could try pecan and cranberry, date and walnut, or tropical fruit. You could also add flaxseeds to the mixture.
- You can increase the amount of nuts and seeds to suit your taste and make it even more nutritious.

> 66 *This is very nice – light and less sugary than other granolas. I like it in the afternoon, when I always get hungry, and struggle with finding healthy snacks that are fairly filling.* 99
> **Becky, 23 weeks pregnant**

Why you should eat oats

Oats have so much to offer. They contain soluble fibre, which helps to regulate blood glucose levels and reduce diabetes risk. Beta-glucan, the particular type of soluble fibre found in oats, also helps reduce blood cholesterol levels, so they are important for heart health too. Oats are also a good source of protein, iron, zinc and B vitamins, including folic acid, which is particularly important in pregnancy. It's better to choose traditional oats rather than instant or quick-cook varieties as they have a lower GI, which means they keep blood sugar levels more stable and are even more beneficial.

French toast and berries

French toast, also known as eggy bread, makes an easy and nutritious breakfast, especially when eaten with berries for a real antioxidant boost.

4 eggs
3 tbsp milk
4 medium slices of granary or wholemeal bread
2 tsp rapeseed oil
175g fresh or defrosted frozen mixed berries (raspberries, strawberries, blackberries, etc.)
2 tbsp honey or maple syrup
½ tsp icing sugar

Preparation time: 5–10 minutes.
Equipment: 1 frying pan and 1 shallow bowl.
Storage: Eat straightaway.
Servings: 2.

- Crack the eggs into the bowl, add the milk and beat with a fork.
- Cut each slice of bread in half diagonally to make two triangles.
- Put some of the bread in the bowl and push it down gently to soak up the egg. Turn the bread over and do the same on the other side.
- Heat one teaspoon of oil in the frying pan, then place four pieces of bread in the pan and fry for 1–2 minutes on each side.
- Place on a warm plate while you repeat with the rest of the bread.
- Drizzle the French toast with honey or syrup, share the berries between the two plates and dust with the icing sugar.

Tip

- For a savoury version serve with grilled tomatoes and mushrooms.

Prune and banana breakfast muffins

These muffins have no added sugar as the prunes and bananas provide plenty of sweetness. If you make a batch for the freezer you can grab one on the way out of the door even if you don't have time to sit down for breakfast.

125g dried prunes
150ml water
2 ripe bananas
1 egg
50ml rapeseed oil
1 tsp vanilla essence
200g plain flour (white, wholemeal or a mixture)
1 tsp baking powder
½ tsp bicarbonate of soda
½ tsp mixed spice

Preparation time: 20 minutes plus 12–15 minutes baking.
Equipment: 1 muffin tin and 1 mixing bowl.
Storage: Airtight container for a few days or freeze.
Servings: 12 muffins.

- Preheat the oven to 200°C (180°C fan)/400°F/gas mark 6. Place paper muffin cases into the muffin tin.
- Place 50g of prunes in a small bowl or a mug with 150ml of tap water. Place in the microwave for 2 minutes on full power, then leave for at least 5 minutes while you prepare the other ingredients.
- Chop the other 75g of prunes.
- Peel the bananas, then place them in the mixing bowl and mash with a potato masher or fork.
- Add the egg, oil and vanilla essence and beat lightly with a fork.
- Mix in the flour, baking powder, bicarbonate of soda, mixed spice and chopped prunes.
- Puree the soaked prunes and mix with the other ingredients.
- Spoon the mixture into the muffin cases and bake for 12–15 minutes, until well risen and spongy to the touch.

Tip

- To make a wheat-free version, replace the flour with 200g spelt flour.

> 66 *As someone who often gets that afternoon 'dip', it was great to pack one of these to keep me going at work, rather than reaching for chocolate or crisps.* 99
> **Magda, 24 weeks pregnant**

Fact or fiction: Prunes are a good cure for constipation

Just mention prunes and someone will have a witty comment about rushing to the toilet. In fact, prunes rarely have an immediate or dramatic effect, but they have been shown in clinical trials to be an effective treatment for mild and moderate constipation. Research has even shown that prunes are more effective than some types of laxatives. Practically all fruit or vegetables will help keep your bowels moving, as they contain fibre, but prunes contain other important substances too. They are rich in sorbitol, which is a type of sugar that is absorbed slowly from the intestines and is known to have a laxative effect, and phenolic compounds including neochlorogenic acid, which also has a laxative effect. Prunes have other valuable nutrients too, including iron, potassium and boron, and research has shown they help slow down glucose absorption and are good for your blood pressure and bone health.

Mushroom kedgeree

Kedgeree is traditionally a breakfast dish that originated in India but it's equally suited to brunch or even lunch or dinner. The mild spices in the rice complement the eggs and mushrooms well.

125g brown basmati rice
2 eggs
2 tsp rapeseed oil
1 small onion
200g mushrooms
2 rounded tsp mild korma paste
¼ lemon, for juice
1 tbsp chopped fresh parsley or 1 tsp dried parsley
salt and freshly ground black pepper

Preparation time: 20–25 minutes.
Equipment: 1 frying pan and 2 small pans.
Storage: Fridge for 24 hours.
Servings: 2.

- Place the rice in a pan with at least 500ml of boiling water. Bring to the boil, then keep at a rolling simmer until cooked, about 12–14 minutes.
- Place the eggs in the second pan and cover with cold water to at least 1cm above the top of the eggs. Bring to the boil. Once you have large bubbles, simmer for 8 minutes.
- Meanwhile, peel and finely dice the onion. Heat the oil in the frying pan and sauté for 2 minutes.
- Slice the mushrooms, then add them to the pan with the onions and cook for a further 5 minutes.
- When the eggs are ready, run them under cold water, then peel off the shell.
- When the rice is cooked, pour it into a sieve, then pour boiling water over it.
- Stir the korma paste into the onion and mushroom mixture, then add the rice and cook for a couple of minutes.
- Add the lemon juice and parsley, then divide the rice between two bowls and place the eggs, cut into quarters, on top. Season with salt and pepper to taste.

Tips

- Kedgeree is traditionally made with smoked haddock. If you'd like to do it this way, then place one or two pieces of fish in a pan, cover with water, bring to the boil and simmer for 5 minutes, then break into chunks and mix with the cooked rice.
- You can also make this with smoked mackerel, which goes very well with eggs.

Lunches, dinners and sides

Carrot and lentil soup

A variation of the ever-popular carrot and coriander soup, this contains lentils for added flavour and slow-release energy.

1 tbsp olive oil
1 onion
4 carrots
½ red pepper
50g red lentils
1 tsp ground coriander
1 bay leaf
600ml stock
salt and pepper

Preparation time: 10 minutes plus 20 minutes simmering.
Equipment: 1 pan.
Storage: Fridge for 24 hours or freeze.
Servings: 3–4.

- Peel and dice the onion. Heat the oil in the pan, add the onion and sweat, without browning, over a low heat for 2–3 minutes with the lid on.
- Peel and slice the carrots, then remove the seeds from the pepper and dice.
- Stir the carrots, red pepper, lentils and coriander in with the onions.
- Add the bay leaf and stock, then bring to the boil and simmer for 20 minutes, until the lentils are cooked and the carrots are tender.
- Remove the bay leaf, then whizz with a stick blender until smooth. Add salt and pepper to taste.

Why you should eat carrots

Carrots are extremely rich in beta-carotene, which is a form of vitamin A, but not the type pregnant women are meant to avoid. The other form, retinol, is found in liver. High intakes can cause birth defects, which is why liver is off the menu in pregnancy. Beta-carotene, on the other hand, should be increased to avoid the risk of vitamin A deficiency, particularly if you're expecting twins or you became pregnant not long after a previous pregnancy. Vitamin A is needed for your baby's skin, eyes and lungs. It also helps ensure you both have a healthy immune system. What's more, beta-carotene is a strong antioxidant and can help ward off pregnancy complications such as pre-eclampsia. Carrots have more beta-carotene than other fruit and vegetables but it's also found in sweet potatoes, pumpkin, butternut squash and cantaloupe melon.

Pea and courgette soup

This vibrant green soup is incredibly quick and easy to cook and makes a perfect lunch.

1 tbsp olive oil
1 onion
2 courgettes
200g frozen peas
1 tbsp chopped fresh basil or ½ tsp dried basil
500ml stock

To serve
salt and pepper
natural yogurt (optional)
fresh chives (optional)

Preparation time: 15 minutes plus 10 minutes simmering.
Equipment: 1 pan.
Storage: Fridge for 24 hours or freeze.
Servings: 4.

- Peel and dice the onion. Heat the oil in the pan, add the onion and sweat, without browning, over a low heat for 2–3 minutes with the lid on.

- Wash the courgettes, chop the ends off, then cut in half lengthways and slice thinly.
- Add the courgettes to the pan and sweat for a further 5 minutes, without browning.
- Add the peas, basil and stock, bring to the boil and simmer with the lid on for 10 minutes, until the vegetables are tender.
- Whizz with a stick blender until smooth or leave it slightly chunky if you prefer.
- Add salt and pepper to taste and serve topped with a spoonful of yogurt and a few chopped chives.

Fact or fiction: Frozen peas are just as healthy as fresh

This is absolutely true. Frozen peas have been found to contain just as much vitamin C as fresh peas. A vast number of studies have compared fresh and frozen fruit and vegetables. Although some have found that blanching vegetables, such as broccoli, before they're frozen means some vitamin C and B vitamins are lost, there isn't much difference overall when looking at the total nutrient content of the resulting cooked vegetables. This is great news if you're trying to eat more vegetables but don't always manage to have fresh ones in the fridge. Stock up on standard frozen veg such as peas, green beans and corn, as well as more exciting ones like spinach, cauliflower or peppers and mixed vegetables so you can throw a handful into stir-fries or pasta sauce.

Mashed chickpeas and avocado

A simple lunchtime dish to serve with sliced tomato. Perfect on granary toast or in warm pitta.

1 x 400g tin chickpeas
1 large avocado
2 tsp lemon juice
1 tsp balsamic vinegar
3 tbsp chopped fresh parsley
½ tsp paprika
salt and pepper

Preparation time: 5 minutes.
Equipment: 1 bowl.
Storage: Fridge for 24 hours.
Servings: 2–3.

- Drain the chickpeas and tip into the bowl.
- Cut the avocado in half, discard the stone and scoop the flesh into the bowl.
- Add the lemon juice, balsamic vinegar, parsley and paprika and mash with a potato masher until the chickpeas are broken but the mixture is still coarse and chunky.
- Add salt and pepper to taste.

Tips

- This also tastes great with a few slices of red onion or some roasted red peppers.
- If you keep this in the fridge overnight, it's fine to eat but will lose its lovely green colour.

Why wholegrain is best

Carbs have received a bad press in recent years but you should actually be getting about half your day's calorie intake from carbohydrates. What's important is the type of carbs you choose – the less refined or processed they are, the better. Wholemeal bread, brown rice and pasta and wholegrain breakfast cereals are nutritionally superior to their white alternatives. They contain more fibre, to keep constipation at bay, and have a lower GI. Not only that but they also contain higher levels of vitamins, minerals and phytochemicals, as these valuable nutrients are found in the outside (brown) layer of the grain. When you eat white versions of carbs, you're keeping the white inside of the grain and throwing away the rest, which is really throwing the baby away with the bathwater. And don't be fooled into thinking French sticks, ciabatta loaves or wraps are better than a sliced white loaf – they're tastier and certainly not off limits, but they're still made from white flour, so it's better if you usually choose wholemeal, granary bread or seeded bread for your daily sandwich.

Greek salad wrap

A delicious wrap made with simple classic ingredients including crumbly feta cheese and black olives.

1 wrap (wholemeal or seeded if possible)
1 tbsp cream cheese (e.g. Philadelphia)
30g feta cheese
1 tomato
2–3cm piece of cucumber
1 tbsp black olives (or green if you prefer)
black pepper

Preparation time: 5 minutes.
Equipment: None.
Storage: Eat straightaway or fridge for 24 hours.
Servings: 1.

- Place the wrap in the oven for a few minutes if you want to eat it warm.
- Chop the cucumber in half lengthways, then slice. Slice the tomato.
- Dice the feta cheese and roughly chop the olives.
- Spread the cream cheese over the wrap, then cover with the tomato, cucumber, feta, olives and some black pepper.
- Roll it up and it's ready.

Why you should make a packed lunch

It's easy to see why sandwich shops are so popular. They're convenient, offer more excitement than the fridge at home and their sandwiches are often tastier. But the satisfying flavour often comes at a price, not just in cash terms but nutritionally too. Their sandwiches are often spread with a thick layer of margarine or full fat mayonnaise, which adds fat and calories before you even get to the filling proper. If you make your own sandwich, you'll save money and be sure of what you're getting. You can leave out the mayonnaise or use a low fat version. You can also pack your sandwich with extra salad. It also means you won't be tempted by the brownie slices at the till and you can go for a walk at lunchtime instead of queuing up at a sandwich shop.

Houmous, spinach and pine nut wrap

Another tasty wrap that tastes good warm or cold.

1 wrap (wholemeal or seeded if possible)
2 tbsp houmous
2 handfuls spinach leaves

½ roasted red pepper (fresh or from a jar)
1 tbsp pine nuts
black pepper

Preparation time: 5 minutes.
Equipment: None.
Storage: Eat straightaway or fridge for 24 hours.
Servings: 1.

- Place the wrap in the oven for a few minutes if you want to eat it warm.
- Put the pine nuts on a baking sheet or piece of foil and put them under the grill for 1–2 minutes until lightly browned.
- Slice the pepper into thin strips.
- Spread the houmous over the wrap, then cover with spinach and scatter with pepper slices and pine nuts. Season with the black pepper.
- Roll up and it's ready to eat.

Why you should wash fruit and vegetables

Perhaps, like many people, you give apples a quick wipe before eating them or run tomatoes under the tap for a second? Well, while you're pregnant it's best to spend a few minutes longer, to make sure you and your baby get all the benefits of fruit and vegetables without picking up a nasty case of food poisoning. All fruit and vegetables, including bags of salad leaves that are labelled as 'washed and ready to eat', should be washed thoroughly before you eat them to avoid the risk of E. coli and listeria. In recent years, outbreaks of food poisoning have been associated with unwashed vegetables, including leeks and potatoes, and bags of watercress. While you're pregnant, changes in your immune system mean you're more susceptible to food poisoning. So it's really important to wash your fruit and vegetables thoroughly – and don't forget your knives and chopping boards too.

Red and white coleslaw with pumpkin seeds

This colourful salad combines crunchy vegetables with a low fat dressing and a generous sprinkling of toasted pumpkin seeds for extra flavour as well as a host of vitamins and minerals.

¼ red cabbage
¼ white cabbage
½ small onion
2 carrots
2 tbsp pumpkin seeds

Dressing
2 tbsp regular or reduced fat mayonnaise
2 tbsp regular or reduced fat salad cream
1 tbsp white wine vinegar
salt and pepper

Preparation time: 15 minutes.
Equipment: 1 bowl.
Storage: Fridge for 24 hours.
Servings: 4–6.

- Peel and finely dice the onion.
- Peel the carrots, wash them, and then grate coarsely.
- Remove the outer leaves of the cabbages and discard, then wash the cabbage and finely shred.
- Put all the vegetables into a large bowl along with the ingredients for the dressing and give everything a good stir.
- Place the pumpkin seeds on a baking tray or a piece of foil and place them under the grill. Toast for a few minutes, until slightly browned and the skin on some has popped.
- Sprinkle the seeds over the coleslaw and serve.

Fact or fiction: Seeds contain omega 3 fatty acids just like oily fish

It's true that many seeds, including flax and pumpkin seeds, contain omega 3 fatty acids, but these are not the same fatty acids found in oily fish. Fish such as salmon and sardines contain long-chain omega 3s, which are important for your baby's brain and eye development (see p129). Seeds, on the other hand, have short-chain omega 3s, which don't provide the same benefits. Our bodies can convert the short-chain omega 3s in seeds and nuts into the beneficial long-chain variety, but we're not very efficient at doing this, and certainly not good enough to get the benefits associated with oily fish. So, if you don't eat oily fish, the only way of getting long-chain omega 3s is by taking a supplement made from fish or seaweed. This doesn't mean that seeds such as flaxseed and pumpkin aren't good for you – they contain polyunsaturated fats, which are much healthier than the saturated fat found in meat products. They're also packed with antioxidants, including vitamin E, as well as being a very good source of zinc, essential for producing healthy new cells.

Watercress and beetroot salad

A refreshing and tasty salad that goes well with pizza, pasta and fish.

1 bag watercress (about 75g)
150g cooked beetroot (vacuum packed but not pickled)
1 small apple (any kind)

Dressing
2 tbsp orange juice
1 tbsp red wine vinegar
1 tsp olive oil
½ tsp wholegrain mustard

Preparation time: 10 minutes.
Equipment: 1 bowl.
Storage: Fridge for 24 hours.
Servings: 2.

- Put all the ingredients for the dressing into a small jug or cup.
- Snip off any tough stalks from the watercress.
- Roughly dice the beetroot into 1–2cm pieces.
- Peel, quarter and core the apple, then cut it into long, thin wedges.
- Mix together the watercress, beetroot and apple, then give the dressing a stir and pour over the salad.

Tip

- This also goes very well in a wrap or pitta with houmous or feta cheese.

Caramelised red onion, beetroot and goats' cheese tart

The sweet onion and beetroot and the tangy goats' cheese complement each other beautifully in this tart, while the polenta base makes a lighter and much healthier alternative to pastry. Good for lunch or a light supper with salad.

400ml vegetable stock
20g Parmesan cheese (or pecorino or similar)
100g polenta (also known as fine corn meal or maize flour)
2 tsp olive oil, plus extra for greasing
1 red onion
2 tbsp balsamic vinegar
175g cooked beetroot (vacuum packed but not pickled)
75g soft goats' cheese

Preparation time: 30 minutes plus 15 minutes baking.
Equipment: 1 pan, 1 frying pan and 1 baking tray.
Storage: Fridge for 24 hours.
Servings: 2.

- Grease the baking tray and grate the Parmesan cheese.
- Bring the stock to the boil in a pan. Pour the polenta into the pan in a steady stream, stirring all the time. Continue to cook for 4–5 minutes, stirring continuously until the polenta thickens and comes away from the sides of the pan.
- Stir in the grated Parmesan, then turn out the mixture onto the centre of the baking tray. Spread out into a circle, about 25cm across, then leave to cool and set.
- Peel, quarter and thinly slice the red onion.
- Heat the oil in a frying pan and gently cook the onion for 5 minutes.
- Preheat the oven to 220°C (200°C fan)/425°F/gas mark 7.
- Add the balsamic vinegar to the onion and cook gently for a further 15 minutes.
- Cut the beetroot into small chunks, add to the onion mixture and heat through.
- Pour the beetroot and onion mixture over the polenta base, crumble the goats' cheese over the top, and bake in the oven for 15 minutes.
- Cut into wedges and serve.

Tip

- Soft goats' cheese is used here rather than chèvre, which is a mould-ripened cheese and has a rind. Soft goats' cheese isn't considered a listeria risk but chèvre is, therefore if you use chèvre make sure the tart is piping hot before serving, to kill any listeria that may be present.

Aubergine parmigiana

A classic Italian dish of baked aubergines and tomatoes topped with mozzarella and Parmesan cheese. This is a much healthier version than the overly cheesy restaurant dish and makes a great lunch with crusty bread, or a perfect side dish with chicken or fish.

1 aubergine
2 tsp olive oil
1 clove garlic
1 x 400g tin chopped tomatoes
1 tsp mixed herbs
¼ tsp mild chilli powder
2 tbsp fresh breadcrumbs (white or wholemeal)
2 tbsp grated Parmesan (or other hard Italian cheese)
25g mozzarella

Preparation time: 15 minutes plus 1 hour baking.
Equipment: 1 baking tray and 1 ovenproof dish.
Storage: Fridge for 24 hours or freeze.
Servings: 2 for lunch or 4 as a side dish.

- Preheat the oven to 190°C (170°C fan)/375°F/gas mark 5.
- Slice the aubergine into 1cm thick slices. Brush the baking tray with one teaspoon of oil, then spread the aubergine slices over the tray and brush them with the remaining oil. Roast in the oven for 30 minutes, turning halfway through.
- Take the aubergine out of the oven and turn the temperature up to 200°C (180°C fan)/400°F/gas mark 6.
- Rub the clove of garlic around the inside of the ovenproof dish. Pour about a third of the tin of tomatoes into the dish and sprinkle with herbs and chilli. Arrange a layer of aubergine in the dish and repeat with another layer of tomato, then aubergine, and finally any remaining tomatoes, herbs and chilli.

- Sprinkle the breadcrumbs and Parmesan over the top and grate or shred the mozzarella into small pieces and place on top.
- Put in the oven for 30 minutes, until the sauce is bubbling and the topping is golden brown.

Tips

- You can also sauté some onion and garlic and add this to the tomato sauce.
- Try adding a few pine nuts and fresh basil on top.

Caponata

This is a Sicilian dish that can be eaten warm or cold. It's made with aubergines and celery in a tomato sauce and it has a slightly sweet–sour flavour from the combination of sugar and red wine vinegar. It goes well with meat, poultry or fish and makes a good pasta sauce.

1 tbsp olive oil
1 red onion
2 sticks celery
1 red pepper
2 cloves garlic
1 aubergine
2 tbsp caster sugar
100ml red wine vinegar
2 tbsp pine nuts
1 x 400g tin chopped tomatoes
1 handful black olives (about 50g)

Preparation time: 45 minutes.
Equipment: 1 deep-sided frying pan.
Storage: Fridge for 24 hours or freeze.
Servings: 4.

- Peel and dice the onion into 1cm pieces. Remove the stem and seeds from the red pepper and dice in the same way. Cut the celery into long strips and dice into pieces about half the size of the onion and pepper.
- Heat one teaspoon of oil in the pan and sauté the onion, pepper, celery and crushed garlic for 10 minutes.
- Meanwhile, cut the aubergine into 1cm cubes.

- Transfer the cooked vegetables to a serving dish. Then heat the remaining oil in the pan and sauté the aubergine for 10 minutes, stirring frequently until soft.
- Transfer the cooked aubergine to the dish with the other vegetables.
- Place the sugar in the pan and heat for about 5 minutes, until starting to lightly brown. Add the vinegar, stir, and leave to cook until the liquid has reduced by about one-third.
- Meanwhile, toast the pine nuts by placing them on a piece of foil and putting them under the grill for 1 minute.
- When the vinegar has reduced, add the tomatoes, vegetables, pine nuts and olives to the pan.
- Stir and heat through, then serve.

Tip

- There are many recipes for caponata and some include capers and sultanas, which you may like to try.

Fact or fiction: If you take a multivitamin it doesn't really matter what you eat

If you don't eat well, then taking a multivitamin and mineral supplement will help you avoid key nutrient deficiencies, but it won't give you all the health benefits of a well balanced diet. For example, diets high in the antioxidant vitamins C and E have been found to be protective against pre-eclampsia in pregnancy. However, when researchers tried giving these vitamins to mums-to-be as a supplement, they didn't have the same effect – in fact, they seemed to cause an unwanted reduction in birth weight. The reason why real foods, especially fruit and vegetables, are so much better could be because of the other beneficial phytochemicals they contain, such as lycopene in tomatoes and anthocyanins in aubergines. There's still plenty to discover about what Mother Nature puts into food, and supplement manufacturers can't possibly offer the same benefits.

Baked courgette and Parmesan crisps

If you're not usually a fan of courgettes, don't be put off – these are very tasty. You can have them as a snack or starter with a dip or as a side dish with anything from Sunday roast to baked potato and beans.

2 medium courgettes (about 300g–350g)
1 tbsp olive oil
20g Parmesan cheese, finely grated
30g breadcrumbs, preferably wholemeal (fresh or dried)
freshly ground black pepper

Preparation time: 5–10 minutes plus 30 minutes baking.
Equipment: 1 baking tray.
Storage: Fridge for 24 hours then reheat under the grill.
Servings: 2–3.

- Preheat the oven to 230°C (210°C fan)/450°F/gas mark 8. Grease the baking tray using some of the oil.
- Cut the ends off the courgettes, then slice into 0.5cm thick rounds.
- Put the slices into a food bag and pour in the oil, then shake to coat the slices.
- Place the breadcrumbs and finely grated cheese into a bowl, add some pepper and mix.
- Place a few slices of courgette into the bowl at a time and press the mixture onto them. Then place them in a single layer on the baking tray.
- Bake in the oven for 25–30 minutes, turning halfway through.

Tips

- Instead of using a bag, you can put the courgette slices in a bowl and drizzle the oil over them if you prefer.
- The Parmesan mixture doesn't stick easily and some slices will end up with more coating than others, but the end result is still delicious.

Easy sweet potato wedges

Sweet potatoes make excellent wedges as they're softer than regular potatoes so don't need parboiling first. Plus, they have a lower GI, which means slow-release energy for both you and your baby.

3 sweet potatoes
2 tsp olive oil or rapeseed oil
¼ tsp paprika

Preparation time: 5 minutes plus 40 minutes baking.
Equipment: 1 baking tray or roasting tin.
Storage: Eat straightaway.
Servings: 2.

- Preheat the oven to 200°C (180°C fan)/400°F/gas mark 6.
- Cut the sweet potatoes into long, chunky wedges.
- Brush the baking tray with one teaspoon of the oil, place the wedges in the tray, sprinkle with the paprika and the rest of the oil and shake gently to toss the wedges around.
- Place in the oven for 40 minutes, turning once or twice while cooking.

Tip

- If you want to spice these up a bit, you can add a little cumin and mild chilli powder.

Leek and celeriac mash

This tasty mash is flavoured with mustard and rosemary and doesn't need the addition of lots of butter or cream for flavour. Excellent with sausages or stews. As celeriac has less than a quarter of the calories found in potatoes, it's a great option if you're finding your weight is increasing more quickly than you'd like.

1 large potato (about 250g–300g)
½ celeriac (about 250g)
1 tsp olive oil or rapeseed oil
1 leek
1 tsp chopped fresh rosemary or ¼ tsp dried rosemary
1 rounded tsp wholegrain mustard

Preparation time: 25 minutes.
Equipment: 1 pan and 1 small frying pan.
Storage: Fridge for 24 hours or freeze.
Servings: 2.

- Peel the potato and chop into chunks. Cover in the pan with water about 4cm above the level of the potatoes and bring to the boil.
- Meanwhile, cut the skin off the celeriac and cut into chunks.

- When the potatoes come to the boil, add the celeriac. Bring back to the boil and simmer for 15–20 minutes, until tender.
- Meanwhile, cut the leek in half lengthways, then slice.
- Heat the oil in the frying pan and sauté the leek for 10 minutes, until soft and slightly browned. Stir in the rosemary and turn off the heat.
- When the potatoes and celeriac are cooked, drain away the water, mash, then stir in the leek and mustard.

Pizza confusion

Pizza is such a simple food, but choosing which one to have when you're pregnant can be far from easy. Any toppings that are properly cooked should be fine. So even though pepperoni, goats' cheese and Brie shouldn't be eaten cold, they're fine on a pizza as cooking will destroy any toxoplasmosis, listeria or other bacteria that could cause food poisoning. If you're thinking of having a pizza topped with Parma ham, be careful as the ham isn't usually cooked but placed on top afterwards, so it could be a food safety risk. Fiorentina pizzas topped with spinach and egg could also be a problem. Some pizzerias may cook the egg completely, but most leave the yolk runny, so these should be avoided in case of salmonella. Once you've considered safety, give health a quick thought too: choose a thin base rather than a thick one and avoid overly cheesy options.

Roast vegetable and goats' cheese pizza

Shop-bought pizzas are often overloaded with cheese and light on the healthier toppings. This pizza, however, has a good helping of tasty roast vegetables combined with tangy goats' cheese. The base isn't a traditional one that needs to be left to rise but an instant one – so your pizza will be on the table in less than half an hour.

Roast vegetables
1 yellow pepper
1 courgette
1 red onion
2 tsp olive oil or rapeseed oil

Base
200g plain flour
pinch salt

3.5g dried yeast (half a 7g sachet)
1 tbsp olive oil, plus extra for greasing
115ml warm water

Topping
200g passata
4 tbsp tomato puree
75g soft goats' cheese

Preparation time: 25 minutes plus 20 minutes baking.
Equipment: 2 baking trays (20cm x 30cm), 1 mixing bowl and 1 small bowl.
Storage: Fridge for 24 hours.
Servings: 2.

- Preheat the oven to 220°C (200°C fan)/425°F/gas mark 7.
- Cut the pepper in half, remove the stalk and seeds and chop into 1–2cm chunks. Cut the courgette into slices no more than 1cm thick. Peel the onion and cut into 1cm wedges.
- Put 1 teaspoon of oil on a baking tray, add all the chopped vegetables and drizzle the other spoonful of oil over the top. Place in the oven for 15 minutes, until the vegetables are nearly soft.
- Grease the other baking tray.
- Mix the passata and tomato puree in a small bowl.
- Place the flour, salt and yeast in a mixing bowl and mix. Make a well in the centre, pour in the oil and water and start to mix with a spoon.
- Using one hand, collect the dough together and place on a floured work surface. Roll out to approximately the size of your baking tray.
- Put the dough on the baking tray.
- When the vegetables have cooked for 15 minutes, turn the oven down to 190°C (170°C fan)/375°F/gas mark 5 and place the base in for 5 minutes.
- Take the trays out of the oven. Spread the tomato sauce over the base, spoon the roast vegetables on top and spread out, then crumble the goats' cheese over the top.
- Return to the oven and cook for a further 15–20 minutes until the edges of the base have browned.

Tip

- You can use a goats' cheese with a rind, such as chèvre, for this recipe, as cooking until it's piping hot will kill any listeria bacteria if they are present. However, you may prefer to use a soft goats' cheese without a rind, which is safe for pregnancy even if it's not cooked.

Lorelei pizza

You may never have had a pizza topped with sardine before, but this was the signature dish of a small, but very popular, pizzeria in Soho for over 25 years.

Base
200g plain flour
pinch salt
3.5g dried yeast (half a 7g sachet)
1 tbsp olive oil, plus extra for greasing
115ml warm water

Topping
200g passata
4 tbsp tomato puree
2 tomatoes
1 x 120g tin sardines in oil
handful black olives
75g mozzarella

Preparation time: 10 minutes plus 20 minutes baking.
Equipment: 1 baking tray (20cm x 30cm), 1 mixing bowl and 1 small bowl.
Storage: Fridge for 24 hours.
Servings: 2.

- Preheat the oven to 190°C (170°C fan)/375°F/gas mark 5. Grease the baking tray.
- Place the flour, salt and yeast in a mixing bowl and mix. Make a well in the centre, pour in the oil and water and start to mix with a spoon.
- Using one hand, collect the dough together and place on a floured work surface. Roll out to approximately the size of your baking tray.
- Put the dough on the baking tray and place in the oven for 5 minutes.
- Meanwhile, mix the passata and tomato puree in a small bowl and slice the tomatoes and mozzarella.
- Drain the sardines, break them in half with a fork and remove the larger central bone.
- Take the pizza base out of the oven, spread the tomato sauce on top followed by the sliced tomatoes and sardines, then the mozzarella and olives.

- Return to the oven and cook for a further 15–20 minutes, until the edges of the base have browned and the cheese has melted.

Tuna and brown rice salad

Brown rice has a lovely nutty taste and adding a soya sauce dressing gives it an even better flavour. This is very simple to prepare and will give you a healthy and satisfying lunch or dinner.

150g raw brown rice or about 300g cooked rice
2 spring onions
½ red pepper (fresh, roasted or pickled)
1 x 140g tin tuna
1 large carrot
2 tbsp frozen soya beans or baby broad beans or peas

Soya sauce dressing
1 tsp sesame oil or olive oil
1 tsp soya sauce
1 tsp lemon juice
1 tsp grated fresh root ginger

Preparation time: 30 minutes boiling rice plus 10 minutes preparing salad.
Equipment: 1 pan.
Storage: Fridge for 24 hours.
Servings: 2.

- Cook the rice according to the instructions on the packet.
- Once the rice is cooked, stir in the frozen soya beans and start to prepare the other ingredients. It's fine if the beans are still frozen as they'll quickly defrost in the hot rice.
- Combine all the ingredients for the dressing and beat with a fork. Use the fork to fluff up the still warm rice and stir in the dressing.
- Finely dice the spring onions and red pepper and peel, then coarsely grate the carrot. Stir into the rice.
- Drain the tinned tuna and stir in.
- Eat warm or cold with a few well-washed salad leaves.

Tips

- Try with other ingredients such as sweetcorn, chopped tomato or cucumber, raisins, pumpkin seeds or cashew nuts.
- Instead of tuna you can use leftover cooked chicken or baked tofu (see p160).

66 This Asian-style salad is packed with flavour and is way more filling than a lunchtime sandwich. The fragrant lemon and ginger is really zingy, and the mix of sesame oil and soy sauce satisfies my savoury cravings! 99
Magda, 24 weeks pregnant

Fact or fiction: Leftover rice causes food poisoning

This isn't true – providing you cool the rice as soon as it's cooked and put it in the fridge within an hour of cooking. However, rice left at room temperature could indeed cause problems. You need to be careful with any food that's left sitting around, for example at barbecues or on buffet tables, but this is especially true for rice. All types of rice contain spores of *Bacillus cereus* bacteria, and if it's left at room temperature these can germinate and multiply. They then produce a toxin that causes food poisoning, including stomach cramps, vomiting and diarrhoea. Reheating cooked rice, even until it's piping hot, won't kill the bacteria if the rice hasn't been cooled properly. If you do cook rice and immediately cool it and put it in the fridge for up to 24 hours, it's fine to eat – either reheated or cold in a salad.

Mediterranean tuna and prawn pasta

Fast, easy and delicious, with prawns and black olives to transform regular tuna pasta into something special.

fusilli, farfalle or other pasta
2 tsp olive oil or rapeseed oil
1 small red onion
½ red pepper
1 clove garlic
1 x 400g tin chopped tomatoes
1 x 160g tin tuna
30g black olives

▌1 tsp dried mixed herbs
▌pinch of chilli powder or dried chilli (optional)
▌100g frozen prawns

Preparation time: 10 minutes plus 10–15 minutes simmering.
Equipment: 1 frying pan and 1 pan for pasta.
Storage: Fridge for 24 hours or freeze.
Servings: 2.

- Cook the pasta according to the instructions on the packet.
- Peel, chop and dice the onion. De-seed the pepper, wash, slice thinly and cut the slices in half.
- Heat the oil in the frying pan and sauté the onion and peppers with the crushed garlic for 5 minutes.
- Add the tomatoes, tuna, olives, herbs and chilli, if using. Stir gently, then bring to the boil and simmer for 5–10 minutes.
- Add the prawns, bring back to the boil and simmer for 1–2 minutes so that the prawns are cooked through.

Fact or fiction: You shouldn't really eat tuna while you're pregnant

Many women think this, and although there's some basis for the belief, it's not true. It's perfectly safe to eat tuna 'in moderation' while you're pregnant and it's actually a very healthy option. The government advises pregnant women to eat no more than two fresh tuna steaks or four 200g tins of tuna a week. This is because tuna has been found to contain very low levels of mercury, which could interfere with the development of your baby's nervous system. The limit for fresh tuna is stricter because it contains far more natural fish oil than tinned tuna. This means that, like other oily fish, it could be contaminated with environmental pollutants and shouldn't be eaten more than twice a week (see p129). Don't let this put you off eating tuna altogether, as it is high in protein and low in fat, as well as being one of the best sources of selenium and vitamins B6 and B12.

Spicy fish tagine

A taste of Morocco with a rich tomato sauce that's flavourful without being hot. It contains plenty of vegetables and goes perfectly with plain couscous and a spoonful of natural yogurt.

▍ 700g firm white fish (e.g. cod, haddock or coley)

▍ *Chermoula (marinade)*
▍ 1 tsp olive oil
▍ 1 clove garlic
▍ 2 tsp ground cumin
▍ 1 tsp ground coriander
▍ 1 tsp ground paprika
▍ juice of 1 lemon

▍ *Tagine*
▍ 1 tbsp olive oil
▍ 1 onion
▍ 2 cloves garlic
▍ 1 tsp ground cumin
▍ 1 tsp ground coriander
▍ 1 tsp ground cinnamon
▍ 1 tsp ground paprika
▍ ½ tsp ground turmeric
▍ 1 green pepper
▍ 1 sweet potato
▍ 250ml vegetable stock
▍ zest of 1 lemon
▍ 2 x 400g tins chopped tomatoes
▍ 50g pimento-stuffed green olives
▍ fresh coriander (optional)

Preparation time: 1 hour.
Equipment: 1 deep-sided frying pan or casserole dish with a lid.
Storage: Fridge for 24 hours or freeze.
Servings: 4.

- In a small bowl, mix together all the ingredients for the chermoula.
- Remove the skin from the fish if it has any. If you have very large fish fillets you might want to cut them so that they're no bigger than 6–8cm.
- Spread the chermoula over the fish and leave it to marinate while you prepare the tagine.
- Dice the onion.
- Heat the oil in the pan and fry the onion and crushed garlic for 5 minutes until soft.

- Meanwhile, cut the pepper in half and remove the seeds, then slice lengthways and cut the slices in half. Peel the sweet potato and dice into 1cm cubes.
- Add the spices to the onion and cook for 2 minutes more, then add the peppers and sweet potato and stir.
- Stir in the stock, then cover and simmer for 10 minutes, until the vegetables are cooked.
- Add the tomatoes, olives and lemon zest and simmer uncovered for 5–10 minutes to reduce the sauce.
- Slide the pieces of fish into the pan, make sure they're covered with a little sauce and cook for about 10 minutes, until the fish is cooked through.
- Scatter with some chopped fresh coriander, if using, and serve.

> 66 *This well-spiced dish is tasty without being hot, and the lemon zest gives it a zingy freshness. It's a relatively easy dinner, despite the long list of ingredients, and is smart enough to serve to friends for a dinner party.* 99
> **Magda, 24 weeks pregnant**

Don't forget white fish

Oily fish, such as salmon and sardines, gets lots of attention for those healthy omega 3s, but white fish, like cod and haddock, is low in fat, contains good-quality protein and provides a host of valuable nutrients. These fish are rich in iodine, which is needed for the development of your baby's nervous system (p38). They're also a good source of selenium, which is an antioxidant that is needed for the development of your baby's immune system. So eating white fish once or twice a week is a very good idea. However, some white fish (sea bass, sea bream, halibut, turbot and dogfish) have been found to contain similar levels of pollutants to oily fish, so these shouldn't be eaten more than twice a week.

Turkey meatballs with warm couscous salad and tzatziki

Lean turkey mince makes delicious light but tasty meatballs. These are mildly spiced and go perfectly with lemon and parsley flavoured couscous salad and refreshing yogurt dip.

Meatballs
500g lean turkey mince
½ small onion
2 cloves garlic
1 tsp paprika
1 tsp ground cumin
1 tbsp fresh parsley
oil for greasing

Couscous salad
6 spring onions
4 tomatoes
handful fresh parsley
300g dried couscous
450ml stock
black pepper

Tzatziki
150g natural yogurt
¼ cucumber

To serve
1 lemon

Preparation time: 30 minutes.
Equipment: 1 baking tray, 1 mixing bowl and 1 pan.
Storage: Eat straightaway or freeze meatballs before cooking.
Servings: 4.

- Preheat the oven to 220°C (200°C fan)/425°F/gas mark 7. Grease the baking tray.
- Peel and finely chop the onion and place in the mixing bowl with the crushed garlic, paprika, cumin and parsley.
- Add the turkey to the bowl and mix all the ingredients using your hands. Take small pieces of the mixture and shape into golf ball-sized meatballs. Place on the greased baking tray. You should have about 16 meatballs.
- Place the meatballs in the oven for 15–20 minutes, turning halfway through and draining away any meat juices that are produced, as these will stop the meatballs baking and browning well.

- Meanwhile, prepare the tzatziki by dicing the cucumber into small pieces and mixing with the yogurt.
- Finely chop the spring onions and parsley and dice the tomatoes.
- Place the couscous in the pan, add the hot stock, stir and leave for 5 minutes with the lid on.
- When the couscous has absorbed all the liquid, add the spring onions, parsley, tomatoes and some black pepper, then stir through using a fork to fluff up the couscous as you go.
- Divide the couscous salad between the four plates, place the meatballs on top and add a good helping of tzatziki. Serve with a wedge of lemon to squeeze over.

Tip

- If you're cooking for fewer than 4 people, put some of the meatballs in the freezer and halve or quarter the ingredients for the couscous and tzatziki.

Lemon and garlic chicken breasts

Grilled chicken is a quick and healthy option, and with this tasty seasoning you can put together a simple midweek meal with just a baked potato and some vegetables.

2 chicken breasts
1 tsp Dijon mustard
½ lemon, for juice and zest
2 cloves garlic
1 tsp olive oil
freshly ground black pepper

Preparation time: 10 minutes plus 15 minutes grilling.
Equipment: 1 baking tray.
Storage: Fridge for 24 hours or freeze.
Servings: 2.

- In a small bowl mix together the mustard, lemon juice and zest, crushed garlic and olive oil.
- Place the chicken breasts between sheets of cling film and beat lightly using a mallet or rolling pin until about 1.5cm thick.
- Preheat the grill to medium hot and line the baking tray with some foil.
- Place the chicken pieces on the baking tray and spread about half the dressing on top.

- Grill for 6–7 minutes, until starting to brown slightly, then turn over, cover with the remaining dressing and grill until the chicken is cooked through and the juices run clear.

Pan-fried pork medallions with leek and apple sauce

A tasty pork dish with creamy leek and apple sauce. Perfect with baked or mashed potatoes and green beans.

250g pork medallions
2 tsp olive oil or rapeseed oil
salt and pepper
1 leek
1 apple
100ml apple juice
4 sage leaves or ½ tsp dried sage, rosemary or mixed herbs
1 clove garlic
3 tbsp cream or reduced fat cream cheese

Preparation time: 25 minutes.
Equipment: 1 large frying pan.
Storage: Fridge for 24 hours or freeze.
Servings: 2.

- Heat the oil in the frying pan and fry the pork, with a little salt and pepper on top, for 3–5 minutes on each side, until nicely browned.
- Meanwhile, cut the leek in half lengthways, wash and slice thinly. Cut the apple into quarters, peel, core and slice thinly. Then finely slice the sage leaves.
- When the pork is cooked, place on a warm plate.
- Put the leek in the pan and cook for 3 minutes, then add the apple and cook for another 3–5 minutes, until tender.
- Add the apple juice to the pan, bring to the boil and cook for a minute or so as you scrape the bottom of the pan to de-glaze.
- Stir in the sage, crushed garlic and cream and return the pork to the pan. Cook for 2–3 minutes more, until the pork is properly cooked through.

Tip

- You may want to cut one of the pieces of pork in half to check that it is cooked through.

Grilled pork skewers

Marinated pork with peppers, mushrooms and courgette makes an easy dinner at home, or cook the skewers on the barbecue for extra flavour. Good with couscous salad (p113) or plain rice and salad.

250g diced pork loin
1 small onion (red or brown)
½ red pepper
4 mushrooms
1 small courgette

Marinade
1 clove garlic
4 sage leaves or rosemary, thyme or parsley
2 tsp olive oil or rapeseed oil
3 tbsp white wine vinegar
2 tbsp Worcestershire sauce
1 tsp soya sauce

Preparation time: 15 minutes plus 1 hour marinating and 10 minutes grilling.
Equipment: 1 bowl and 1 baking tray.
Storage: Fridge for 24 hours.
Servings: 2.

- Crush the garlic into a bowl, chop the sage and mix with all the other marinade ingredients. Stir in the diced pork, cover with cling film and leave in the fridge for at least an hour.
- When the meat has marinated, chop the onion and pepper into large chunks, cut the mushrooms in half and slice the courgette into 1cm slices.
- Thread the pork and vegetables onto four metal skewers and place on a baking tray. Pour any remaining marinade over the top.
- Place under a medium hot grill for 10 minutes, turning occasionally, until the meat is cooked through and the vegetables are browning.

Tip

- If you use wooden skewers, make sure you soak them for at least half an hour beforehand, otherwise they can burn.

Beef stroganoff

An update of the classic Russian dish of steak and mushrooms in a creamy sauce. Serve with rice, pasta or mash.

1 rump or sirloin steak
salt and freshly ground black pepper
½ tsp paprika
1 tbsp rapeseed oil
1 onion
2 cloves garlic
150g mushrooms
150ml stock
1 tsp cornflour mixed with 1 tbsp cold water
2 rounded tbsp natural yogurt
1 tbsp chopped fresh parsley (optional)

Preparation time: 25 minutes.
Equipment: 1 deep-sided frying pan.
Storage: Fridge for 24 hours or freeze.
Servings: 2.

- Trim the fat off the steak and cut slightly diagonally into 0.5 1cm thick strips. Cover with a little salt and pepper and the paprika.
- Peel and dice the onion, then heat 2 teaspoons of the oil in the frying pan and sauté the onion for 2 minutes.
- Slice the mushrooms and add them to the pan, along with the garlic, and cook for 5 minutes, until soft and starting to brown nicely. Then transfer to a plate.
- Add the remaining oil to the pan and fry the steak for about 2 minutes to brown. Then transfer to the plate.
- Slowly add the stock to the pan, stirring to combine any brown bits from the bottom of the pan. Bring to the boil, then add the cornflour and water mixture and stir for a minute to thicken.
- Put the steak and mushroom mixture back in the pan along with the yogurt and warm through. Check that the steak is cooked, then turn off the heat and sprinkle with parsley, if using.

Desserts and snacks

Apple and prune crumble with sesame oat topping

This is lovely and sweet and the topping has a mild caramel-like flavour. Delicious on its own or with custard or vanilla ice cream.

4 eating apples
100g pitted prunes
50ml water
½ tsp ground cinnamon
50g oats
50g wholemeal flour
30g demerara sugar
2 tbsp sesame seeds
50ml rapeseed oil

Preparation time: 15 minutes plus 30 minutes baking.
Equipment: 1 pan, 1 mixing bowl and 1 ovenproof dish.
Storage: Fridge for 1–2 days or freeze.
Servings: 4–6.

- Preheat the oven to 200°C (180°C fan)/400°F/gas mark 6.
- Quarter the apples, then peel and core them and cut into chunks.
- Put the apple chunks, prunes, cinnamon and water in a pan, bring to the boil and simmer for 5 minutes, until the apple is soft.
- Meanwhile, mix the oats, flour, sugar, sesame seeds and oil in a bowl.
- Transfer the apple and prune mixture to an ovenproof dish and spoon over the topping.
- Place in the oven for 30 minutes, until nicely browned.

Honey plums

Warm, honey-sweetened plums with natural yogurt or a scoop of your favourite ice cream.

4 plums
2 tbsp orange juice
1 tbsp honey

To serve
200g yogurt or 2 scoops of ice cream
1 tbsp flaked almonds

Preparation time: 5 minutes plus 5 minutes simmering.
Equipment: 1 pan.
Storage: Eat straightaway.
Servings: 2.

- Cut the plums in half and remove the stones, then slice into thin wedges.
- Heat the orange juice and honey in the pan until bubbling.
- Add the sliced plums to the pan and stir. When it starts to bubble again, put the lid on and leave to cook for 5 minutes, stirring occasionally. The plums should be soft but not mushy.
- Turn off the heat and eat straightaway or leave to sit while you eat your main course and serve slightly warm.
- Put into bowls with yogurt or ice cream on top and a sprinkle of flaked almonds.

Chocolate mousse

A rich chocolate mousse that you can enjoy without worrying, as it gets its light airiness from marshmallows instead of raw eggs.

40g dark chocolate (70% cocoa solids)
45g mini marshmallows
½ tsp vanilla essence
75ml milk
75ml double cream

Preparation time: 15 minutes plus at least 30 minutes in the fridge.
Equipment: 1 pan and 1 bowl.
Storage: Fridge for 24 hours.
Servings: 2.

- Break up the chocolate and put it in a pan with the marshmallows, vanilla essence and milk.
- Gently warm the mixture, stirring all the time until the chocolate and marshmallows have melted and all the ingredients are mixed together. Take the pan off the heat and leave to cool.

- Pour the cream into a bowl and whip until it forms soft peaks.
- Add the cooled chocolate mixture to the cream and give it a quick whisk to combine.
- Pour into two ramekins, wine glasses or other dishes, cover with cling film and place in the fridge for at least 30 minutes to set.

Tips

- This tastes delicious with fresh strawberries or raspberries.
- To cool the chocolate mixture quicker, fill the sink with a little cold water and put the pan in it.

Tiramisu

Tiramisu is usually off the menu during pregnancy as it contains alcohol and semi-cooked eggs, never mind the caffeine in the espresso. Although this version couldn't claim to be a health food, it tastes wonderful and you can eat it without any safety worries.

80g sponge fingers
1 tsp instant coffee (regular or decaffeinated)
2 tsp cocoa powder
150ml boiling water
100g mascarpone cheese
15g custard powder
15g sugar
250ml milk
50g half-fat squirty cream or 150ml whipped double cream
15g grated dark chocolate

Preparation time: 20 minutes plus 1 hour chilling.
Equipment: 1 glass dish.
Storage: Fridge for 2 days.
Servings: 4.

- Place the coffee and 1 teaspoon of cocoa into a bowl with 150ml of boiling water, stir and leave to cool slightly.
- Put the custard powder and sugar in a microwave-safe bowl or jug. Make a smooth paste with a little of the milk, then add the rest and heat in the microwave for about 3 minutes until thick. Stir well and leave to cool slightly.

- Place a few sponge fingers in the coffee mixture at a time, leave for a few seconds, turn over, and then place in the bottom of the glass dish. Do this with about half the fingers.
- Beat the mascarpone cheese into the custard using a wire bulb whisk or fork, then pour about half the mixture over the sponge fingers.
- Sprinkle half a teaspoon of cocoa powder on top, then repeat the process with another layer of coffee-soaked fingers, followed by the rest of the custard mixture and more cocoa powder.
- Cover the dish and leave it in the fridge for at least 1 hour.
- Before serving, squirt cream all over the top of the dessert and sprinkle on the grated chocolate.

Tips

- For a more indulgent dessert, use full fat milk to make the custard or buy ready-made custard and use double cream instead of squirty cream.
- If you buy tiramisu from a supermarket, it should be safe to eat as it will be made with pasteurised egg and very little coffee or alcohol. If you're eating at a friend's house or in a restaurant, however, it's best to ask.

Raspberry and yogurt muffins

You don't need as much sugar to make these as you would with traditional muffins as they get all the flavour they need from juicy raspberries and tangy yogurt.

125g wholemeal flour
125g plain flour
1 tbsp baking powder
75g soft brown sugar
100ml rapeseed oil
2 eggs
200g low fat natural yogurt
225g frozen or fresh raspberries

Preparation time: 15 minutes plus 30 minutes baking.
Equipment: 1 bun or muffin tray and 1 large mixing bowl.
Storage: Airtight container for a few days or freeze.
Servings: 10 muffins.

- Preheat the oven to 200°C (180°C fan)/400°F/gas mark 6. Fill your muffin tray with paper cases.
- Place the flour, baking powder and sugar in a mixing bowl and mix.
- Place the oil, yogurt and eggs in a measuring jug and beat lightly.
- Pour the oil mixture into the bowl and fold into the flour and sugar.
- Add the raspberries and gently stir to combine all the ingredients. Don't worry if the raspberries are still frozen.
- Spoon the mixture into the cake cases and bake for 25–30 minutes, until well risen and nicely browned.

> 66 *These are easy to make and taste really good – not as sweet as most muffins.* 99
> Becky, 23 weeks pregnant

Why you should eat raspberries

You should eat raspberries for the same reason you should have blueberries, blackberries and any other kind of berry. They're delicious and very healthy. Particular berries may be the latest 'superfood' and be priced accordingly, but all berries offer a host of health benefits. They're also low in calories, which makes them perfect for satisfying sweet cravings without piling on the pounds. They contain a range of phytochemicals, which provide them with their vibrant colours and make them especially rich sources of antioxidants. While antioxidants are valuable for everyone, giving protection against heart disease and cancer, they're even more important for pregnant women. Research suggests that eating antioxidant-rich foods in pregnancy helps protect against pre-eclampsia and reduces the chances of your baby developing allergies.

Wheat-free chocolate cake

A great recipe for those who can't eat wheat and for anyone who loves chocolate cake. This is rich and super-chocolaty and you'd never guess it was made of beans if you hadn't made it yourself.

1 x 400g tin adzuki beans or black beans or kidney beans
60g cocoa powder
2 tbsp rapeseed oil
1 tbsp vanilla essence

1 tsp baking powder
½ tsp bicarbonate of soda
100g caster sugar
4 eggs
1 tsp icing sugar for dusting

Preparation time: 15 minutes plus 30 minutes baking.
Equipment: 1 blender or mixing bowl and hand-held blender, and a loose-based cake tin (23cm diameter).
Storage: Airtight container for a few days or freeze
Servings: 1 large cake (about 12 slices).

- Preheat the oven to 180°C (160°C fan)/350°F/gas mark 4. Grease the cake tin and line the bottom with greaseproof paper.
- Drain the beans and place in the bowl, sieve the cocoa powder into the bowl too, then add all the remaining ingredients, apart from the icing sugar.
- Blend all the ingredients together to form a smooth, runny batter.
- Pour the batter into the cake tin and bake for about 30 minutes until a skewer inserted in the centre comes out dry.
- Leave to cool completely before removing from the tin.
- Dust with icing sugar.

Tip

- This cake is delicious as it is with a cup of tea, or serve with mixed berries and crème fraîche or ice cream.

> 66 *Even my self-confessed chocaholic friend loved this cake, and could hardly believe it was made with beans. It's delicious with a scoop of vanilla frozen yogurt – and feels very virtuous!* 99
> **Magda, 24 weeks pregnant**

Second trimester meal planner

Although you don't need to follow a meal plan while you're pregnant, the one laid out here shows what a healthy diet for the second trimester looks like. It includes plenty of fruit and vegetables, some starchy carbohydrate-rich foods with each meal, and a few snack foods too.

This meal plan meets the requirements for energy, protein, potassium, calcium, magnesium, phosphorus, iron, copper, zinc, chloride, selenium, iodine, thiamin, riboflavin, niacin and vitamins A, B6, B12, C and E.

To meet all the nutrient requirements for this stage of pregnancy, you would also need to take a supplement containing 10µg vitamin D (see p9) and have plenty of water or other drinks.

Day 1

Breakfast: Carrot cake porridge (p63)
Lunch: Greek salad wrap (p72), a banana
Dinner: Lemon and garlic chicken breast (p92), baked potato with cottage cheese, mixed salad, honey plums (p96) with crème fraîche
Snacks: Malt loaf, plain popcorn

Day 2

Breakfast: Granary toast, scrambled eggs and grilled tomato
Lunch: Wholemeal pitta, houmous, avocado, cucumber and carrot sticks
Dinner: Roast vegetable and goats' cheese pizza (p83), watercress and beetroot salad (p76)
Snacks: Prune and banana breakfast muffin (p66), an apple

Day 3

Breakfast: Branflakes with sliced strawberries
Lunch: Wholemeal toast, baked beans, an orange
Dinner: Tuna and brown rice salad (p86), strawberries and ice cream
Snacks: Mixed nuts and raisins, a packet of crisps

Day 4

Breakfast: Prune and banana breakfast muffins (p66), a fruit yogurt
Lunch: Baked potato with tuna and sweetcorn, mixed salad
Dinner: Beef stroganoff (p95), rice, fruit salad
Snacks: Muesli

Day 5

Breakfast: 2 Weetabix with milk, slice of granary toast with peanut butter
Lunch: Pea and courgette soup (p70), ciabatta with tomato and mozzarella
Dinner: Grilled salmon steak, easy sweet potato wedges (p81), corn on the cob, tomato and onion salad, chocolate mousse (p97)
Snacks: Toast with yeast extract, a peach

Day 6

Breakfast: Porridge, grapefruit
Lunch: Caramelised red onion, beetroot and goats' cheese tart (p77), green salad
Dinner: Spaghetti with pesto, mixed salad, a yogurt
Snacks: Dried prunes, oat biscuits, toast and yeast extract

Day 7

Breakfast: Honey nut granola (p64), raspberries
Lunch: Chicken salad sandwich, a yogurt drink
Dinner: Grilled pork skewers (p94), rice, red and white coleslaw (p74), wheat-free chocolate cake (p100) with raspberries
Snacks: Carrot and cucumber sticks with houmous, fig roll biscuits

4 The third trimester

In the last months of pregnancy your baby is growing rapidly and her senses are becoming more sophisticated. By week 31 she'll be able to hear your voice, see the difference between light and dark and also taste what you've been eating. It's exciting to think you'll soon be meeting your baby, but if you're suffering from sleepless nights, an aching back or other problems, then the final weeks may seem to drag on. In the meantime, both you and your baby have plenty to do in preparation for the birth – a baby's weight trebles in the last trimester, her brain and skeleton grow rapidly, and her lungs and other organs mature. Your baby will also be laying down fat to provide stores for the first days of life on the outside.

All that growth inevitably requires extra nutrients. Some of these needs are met by adaptations your body has already made. For example, you will have been accumulating additional long-chain omega 3s ready to fuel the rapid brain growth that occurs in these last months. Your digestive system will also adapt to absorb about 50% more iron than it did at the beginning of your pregnancy. While these changes go some way to meeting your baby's high nutrient requirements, healthy eating is still vital. Not only is it important for your baby's growth and development, but it will keep you in good health and prepare you for labour.

Although there was no need to increase your energy intake earlier in pregnancy, you are advised to eat an additional 200 calories per day during this final trimester. These extra calories should come from healthy foods that will supply you with the right nutrients. This section of the book contains several snack recipes that fit the bill, as well as plenty of nutrient-dense meals to make it easy for you to meet your daily requirements.

200 calorie pregnancy snacks

- A banana and a small pot of low fat yogurt
- A small bowl of muesli (40g) with semi-skimmed milk
- A portion of chocolate popcorn (p143)
- A slice of wholemeal toast with houmous and carrot sticks
- Three oat cakes with very thinly sliced Cheddar
- 40g bag of mixed nuts and raisins
- A slice of granary toast and one scrambled egg
- A thick slice of malt loaf and an apple
- One wholemeal pitta filled with cream cheese and sliced tomato

You may notice you're feeling hotter than usual as your baby acts as a personal radiator, and it's important to drink plenty of water. With that raised temperature, it's easier to overheat, so it's best to keep out of the midday sun and have a cold drink to hand. Keeping well hydrated will also help you avoid becoming constipated, or ease symptoms if you're already suffering. When possible, drink between meals rather than having lots to drink at mealtimes, otherwise it can make you feel overly full and increase the chances of heartburn. This is a common problem as your bump expands, but making small changes to the way you eat can help (p145).

You'll probably find yourself slowing down even more at this stage. While it's good to walk and get some fresh air every day, as well as regular gentle exercise, you shouldn't push yourself too much or overdo the activities. It's normal to feel breathless more easily, as your growing bump leaves less room for your lungs. In the last weeks of pregnancy, when your baby's head is likely to become engaged in preparation for birth, you should find that both breathlessness and heartburn ease because there is now more room for your lungs and stomach. As your joints relax in preparation for making the birth easier, it also becomes easier for you to get an injury or strain. This is another reason to make sure you exercise carefully. It also means caution is needed when lifting anything heavy.

How to improve your sleep

- Avoid all caffeine in the afternoon and evening.
- Have a milky drink before bed (p145).
- Turn off all computers, smart phones, etc. an hour before bed.
- Have a warm bath with lavender.
- Make yourself as comfortable as possible with extra pillows.

As this trimester progresses, anyone working will no doubt be longing to start their maternity leave. If you already have children, see if you can still get some time to yourself. Make the most of this time to rest and put your feet up while you have the chance. As you prepare for your baby's arrival, you'll probably be thinking about clothes and nappies and other essentials. But now is also the time to stock up your kitchen cupboards with essentials such as pasta and tins of tomatoes, and put some meals in the freezer ready for those busy early days with the new baby. You may think it won't be that difficult, as you'll be at home all day and maybe also have a partner helping out some of the time, but you'll be surprised at how much time and how many hands it takes to care for one little baby. Many of the recipes in this section are designed with this in mind. Stews, casseroles and curries are ideal for freezing and the recipes are made to feed four people, so, depending on the size of your family, you may be able to eat half now and put the rest in the freezer for another day.

Labour bag snacks

When you pack your labour bag to take to the hospital, or get things ready for a home birth, don't forget about snacks. Many women find they don't want anything to eat at that stage, but others find they really need something to keep their energy levels up, so it's good to be prepared.

Ideal snacks to pack include:

- mini cartons of juice
- a bottle of water and a straw
- glucose tablets or jelly sweets
- oatcakes, cereal bars or breakfast bars (good for afterwards).

You can pack biscuits or chocolate or anything you like, really – and don't forget your birthing partner. Some report that it can be quite a tiring and hungry job – poor things!

As your due date approaches, or comes and goes, you'll be advised by friends to have a hot curry, eat some pineapple or try something else. These are very unlikely to bring on labour if it wasn't about to start anyway, but there are several curry recipes in this section for you to enjoy (pp121, 122 and 132). Instead of wishing the time away, use the brief respite to relax, and if your freezer is already stocked up with dinners, then bake some wholemeal fig muffins (p108) or Cheddar scones (p179) to freeze too – you'll be glad of them later!

Breakfasts

Breakfast bruschetta

A tasty breakfast of toasted granary rolls topped with creamy spinach, fried mushrooms and fluffy scrambled eggs. It also makes a good lunch.

2 granary rolls or wholemeal muffins or thick slices of bread
3 eggs
2 tbsp milk
1 tsp olive oil or rapeseed oil
4 mushrooms
125g frozen spinach
1 tbsp cream cheese
sprinkle of nutmeg
black pepper

Preparation time: 15 minutes.
Equipment: 1 frying pan.
Storage: Eat straightaway.
Servings: 2.

- Beat the eggs and milk in a small bowl or mug.
- Slice the mushrooms. Heat the oil in the frying pan and fry the mushrooms for 3–4 minutes, until nicely browned.
- Meanwhile place the spinach in the microwave for 3–4 minutes and put the bread or rolls in the toaster.
- When the mushrooms are ready, add the egg mixture, leave for a minute, then stir until set and no runny egg remains.
- Mix the cream cheese and nutmeg into the hot spinach.

- Take two warm plates, put a roll or a slice of toast on each, and spread the spinach mixture on top followed by the egg and mushroom and some black pepper.

Wholemeal fig muffins

These make a good breakfast if you're on the go and don't have time to sit down. To make a really well balanced meal, have them with some fresh fruit and yogurt.

200g wholemeal flour
150g plain flour
5 tsp baking powder
100g demerara sugar
200g dried figs
2 eggs
250ml milk
125ml rapeseed oil
2 tbsp oats

Preparation time: 15 minutes plus 20 minutes baking.
Equipment: 1 muffin tin and 1 mixing bowl.
Storage: Airtight container for a few days or freeze.
Servings: 12 large muffins.

- Preheat the oven to 200°C (180°C fan)/400°F/gas mark 6. Place paper cases into the muffin tin.
- In the mixing bowl, combine the flours, baking powder and sugar.
- Coarsely chop the figs, discarding any tough stalks, and combine with the dry ingredients in the bowl.
- Make a well in the centre and crack the eggs into it. Beat lightly, then add the oil and milk and beat again.
- Gently combine all the ingredients, being careful not to over-mix and mush the figs.
- Spoon the muffin mixture into the paper cases and sprinkle the oats over the top. Bake for 20 minutes, until well risen and spongy to the touch.

Apple, prune and almond bircher muesli

This is like a summery version of porridge. It takes only 5 minutes to mix together the ingredients the night before, then you can wake up to a tasty and satisfying breakfast. This version is soaked in orange juice, which gives it a more refreshing taste and increases iron absorption, but you can use apple juice, water or milk instead.

100g porridge oats
15g flaked almonds
60g prunes
1 apple
250ml orange juice
50ml water

To serve
milk and/or natural yogurt or soya equivalent

Preparation time: 5–10 minutes.
Equipment: An airtight container or bowl and cling film.
Storage: Fridge for 24 hours.
Servings: 2.

- Place the oats and almonds in the container.
- Chop the prunes into the mixture.
- Cut the apple into quarters, remove the core, then grate into the mixture.
- Add the orange juice and water, give it a stir, cover with cling film and place in the fridge.
- In the morning, give it another stir, spoon into cereal bowls and serve with milk and/or yogurt.

Tips

- This basic recipe can be halved for one person or increased for more than two.
- Adjust according to taste by using other dried fruits and nuts.
- You can also add sliced banana or strawberry in the morning or other berries.
- If you don't have time to make this in advance, you can just leave it to soak for 5 minutes and it will still taste good.

Why you should have a good iron intake

You need iron to make healthy red blood cells to carry oxygen around your body. It's also needed for the liver and nervous system to function properly, and if your iron levels are low you may feel tired, faint, irritable and unable to concentrate. Anaemia, or iron deficiency, is also associated with feeling low or depressed, and is fairly common in pregnancy. If your blood tests show you are anaemic, you will need iron supplements, but otherwise you should try to get plenty of iron from the foods you eat. Unless you have been told you are anaemic, it's not considered beneficial to take an iron supplement, and it may actually be harmful. The right foods will ensure your baby is born with good iron stores and that you have reserves ready to cope with blood loss during labour. Good sources of iron include breakfast cereals with added iron, bread, meat, poultry, fish, lentils and dried fruit. When you have a meal, think about what you have to drink – a cup of tea will reduce the amount of iron you absorb from your food, whereas a glass of orange juice will increase iron absorption.

Blueberry pancakes

These light and fluffy pancakes make a tasty weekend breakfast and also provide the fibre, calcium and antioxidants that you need.

125g wholemeal flour
1 tsp baking powder
1 egg
100g regular or low fat natural yogurt
100ml milk
200g blueberries
1 tsp rapeseed oil

To serve
extra yogurt
a little maple syrup or honey

Preparation time: 15 minutes.
Equipment: 1 frying pan and 1 mixing bowl or blender.
Storage: Fridge for 24 hours or freeze.
Servings: 2 (6 pancakes).

- Place the flour, baking powder, egg, yogurt and milk in a blender or in a bowl and whisk with a fork, wire whisk or hand-held blender.
- Stir in 75g of blueberries.
- Heat the oil in the frying pan, then pour in about 2 tablespoonfuls of the mixture to make each pancake. You should be able to make 3–4 pancakes at a time.
- Once the edges of the pancake look dry and bubbles start to appear on the surface, flip the pancake over. Each side will need 1–2 minutes to cook.
- Serve with a drizzle of syrup or honey and some yogurt on the side, along with the rest of the blueberries.

Tips

- You can also add a little lemon zest to the batter for a sharper flavour.
- Half the wholemeal flour can be replaced with plain flour if you prefer.
- The pancakes also taste good with blueberry compote.
- If you freeze the pancakes, reheat them under the grill.

Lunches, dinners and sides

Italian fish soup

Fennel and tomato are key ingredients in Italian fish soup and give it a distinctive Mediterranean taste. This simple recipe is perfect as it is but you can add to it with fresh herbs and seafood such as king prawns or scallops.

2 fillets of fish (see tips below)
1 tbsp olive oil
1 small onion
1 bulb of fennel
2 cloves garlic
1 x 400g tin chopped tomatoes
1 bay leaf
350ml fish or vegetable stock
2 tbsp chopped fresh parsley or 2 tsp dried parsley

Preparation time: 40 minutes.
Equipment: 1 large pan and a hand-held blender.
Storage: Fridge for 24 hours.
Servings: 2–4.

- Peel and dice the onion and dice the fennel into 1–2cm pieces.
- Heat the oil in the pan and sauté the onion and fennel for 5 minutes. Add the crushed garlic and cook for 2 minutes more.
- Add the tomato, bay leaf, stock and parsley, bring to the boil and simmer for 10 minutes, until the vegetables are tender.
- Meanwhile, cut the fish into bite-sized chunks.
- Remove the bay leaf and puree the tomato sauce until it is completely smooth, or slightly chunky if you prefer.
- Add the fish and cook for about 5 minutes, until it is cooked through.

Tips

- This would traditionally be made with white fish but it works well with one fillet of oily fish, such as salmon, and one piece of white fish, like cod or haddock.
- This makes a good dinner for two with some bread or leftover potatoes added in, or as lunch for up to four people.

Spinach and pumpkin seed salad with honey balsamic dressing

This is a beautifully colourful salad that's brimming with flavour. It's easy to get your 5-a-day when it tastes this good.

75g baby spinach leaves
1 large carrot
6–8 cherry tomatoes
1 tbsp pumpkin seeds
1 tbsp sunflower seeds

Dressing
2 tsp runny honey
1 tbsp balsamic vinegar
1 tsp sesame oil or olive oil

Preparation time: 10 minutes.
Equipment: 1 bowl.
Storage: Fridge for 24 hours.
Servings: 2.

- Put the seeds onto a small piece of aluminium foil on your grill tray and toast under a medium hot grill for 2–3 minutes.
- Peel and grate the carrot and cut the tomatoes in half, then toss them in the bowl along with the spinach leaves.
- Combine the ingredients for the dressing in a small cup or jug and pour over the salad.
- Sprinkle on the seeds and serve.

Tip

- Alternatively, you can make a honey and mustard dressing with 2 tsp honey, 1 tbsp white wine or cider vinegar, 1 tsp olive oil and ½ tsp wholegrain mustard.

Fact or fiction: Spinach is a good source of iron

Spinach certainly contains iron, but eating spinach won't actually help you get the iron you need, as spinach is rich in oxalic acid, which binds tightly to the iron so that it can't be absorbed by the body. So this one is fiction. However, spinach is an excellent source of vitamin E, containing more than three times as much as lettuce or cabbage. This means it will help with the development of your baby's nervous system and could help protect her from developing asthma or other allergies. Spinach also contains more calcium, potassium, carotene and folate than similar vegetables, making it an excellent vitamin and mineral booster for pregnancy.

Mediterranean couscous salad

Ripe tomatoes, artichoke hearts and black olives are combined with lemon and herb couscous to make a wonderful Mediterranean salad. Including mixed beans in the dish and crumbling feta cheese on top adds contrast to the flavours and makes it an ideal all-in-one dish for a quick lunch at home or a packed lunch at work.

100g couscous
1 tsp dried basil or 1 tbsp fresh basil
1 tsp mixed dried herbs or 1 tbsp fresh rosemary, parsley or thyme
150ml boiling water
½ tin artichoke hearts or about 120g from a jar
2 tbsp pitted black olives
handful of ripe tomatoes (e.g. vine-ripened or cherry plum tomatoes)

75g roasted red pepper from a jar
1 x 400g tin mixed bean salad in water or cannellini, borlotti, butter or other beans
2 tsp lemon juice
1 tsp balsamic vinegar
2 tsp olive oil
40g feta cheese

Preparation time: 10–15 minutes.
Equipment: 1 large bowl.
Storage: Fridge for 24 hours.
Servings: 2.

- Place the couscous in the bowl, stir in the herbs and cover with boiling water. Leave until the water has been absorbed.
- Cut the artichoke hearts into quarters. Slice the olives and chop the tomatoes and peppers.
- Add the lemon juice, balsamic vinegar and olive oil to the couscous (no need to wait for it to cool), then stir in the chopped vegetables and the drained beans.
- Crumble the feta cheese over the top.

Thai-style carrot and orange slaw

A light and refreshing salad made with oranges and spring onions and tossed in a peanut, lime and honey dressing.

1 large carrot
100g cabbage (green, white or sweetheart)
1 orange
3 spring onions

Dressing
2 heaped tsp peanut butter (smooth or crunchy)
1 tbsp rice wine vinegar or cider vinegar
1 tsp honey
½ tsp reduced salt soya sauce
1 tsp lime juice

Preparation time: 10 minutes.
Equipment: 1 bowl.
Storage: Eat straightaway or fridge for 24 hours.
Servings: 2.

- Peel and coarsely grate the carrot.
- Discard the outer leaves of the cabbage and shred finely.
- Cut the peel off the orange, then chop into small pieces.
- Slice the spring onion, including most of the green. Mix the vegetables and orange together in the bowl.
- In a small bowl or cup, combine all the ingredients for the dressing using a fork.
- Pour the dressing over the salad and stir.

> 66 *The Thai slaw was extremely easy to make and the ingredients were nice and cheap, though neither my husband nor I like raw onions so we left those out. It was tasty and satisfying but also felt very wholesome to eat. We'll be having it again.* 99
> **Corey, 34 weeks pregnant (and mum to Marcus, 18 months)**

Fact or fiction: If you eat peanuts your baby is more likely to get an allergy

Ten years ago, scientists weren't really sure, so pregnant women were advised to avoid nuts just in case. However, research has now shown this isn't the case. Avoiding peanuts doesn't reduce your baby's risk of developing allergies, and it may actually increase it. The same goes for other foods that are more likely to cause allergies, such as milk, wheat, fish and soya. So, unless you are allergic to any particular food yourself, there is no benefit in avoiding it. Some experts believe the best way of protecting your baby from allergies is actually to eat as wide a range of foods as possible during pregnancy. The results of some research studies also suggest that eating a diet rich in antioxidants is important as it helps your baby develop a healthy immune system, while other research suggests that long-chain omega 3 fatty acids or probiotics and prebiotics may be protective. There isn't enough evidence to prove that any particular strategy will protect your baby from allergies, but eating a varied and healthy diet should cover all these bases.

Indian salad

This goes well with just about any curry or Indian-style dish and is an easy way to add an extra portion of vegetables to your diet.

5cm piece of cucumber
1 large tomato
¼ onion
2 tbsp fresh coriander (optional)

Dressing
2 rounded tbsp low fat natural yogurt
¼ tsp Dijon mustard
1 tsp white wine vinegar
pinch ground cumin

Preparation time: 5 minutes.
Equipment: 1 bowl.
Storage: Eat straightaway or fridge for 24 hours.
Servings: 2.

- Peel and finely dice the onion and put in a bowl. Add the coriander (if using).
- Dice the tomato and cucumber into 1cm pieces and add them to the onion. There is no need to remove the cucumber skin unless it is particularly thick.
- In a small bowl or cup, combine all the ingredients for the dressing.
- Pour the dressing over the salad and stir.

Mediterranean-style stuffed courgettes

Courgette boats filled with a mixture of tomato, red pesto and cheese – perfect for a vegetarian lunch with some crusty bread and salad or as a side dish with meat or fish.

2 courgettes
oil for greasing
50g wholemeal or granary breadcrumbs
2 medium tomatoes
2 tsp red pesto
1 egg
40g mozzarella or Cheddar

Preparation time: 20 minutes plus 15–20 minutes baking.
Equipment: 1 baking tray and 1 bowl.
Storage: Eat straightaway or fridge for 24 hours.
Servings: 2 as a main course.

- Preheat the oven to 220°C (200°C fan)/425°F/gas mark 7. Grease the baking tray.
- Cut the courgettes in half lengthways and run a teaspoon down the cut sides to scoop out the soft centre containing the seeds.
- Place the courgettes on the baking tray, cut side up, and bake for 15 minutes.
- Meanwhile, prepare the breadcrumbs in a food processor and dice the tomatoes into pieces no larger than 1cm.
- Place the breadcrumbs, chopped tomatoes, pesto and egg in a bowl, plus either shredded mozzarella or grated Cheddar. Mix well with a fork so that all the ingredients are combined thoroughly.
- When the courgettes are ready, spoon the stuffing mixture down the centre and return to the oven for 15–20 minutes, until the top is crispy.

Braised red cabbage

Red cabbage takes a long time to cook but it's worth it because it's packed with beneficial phytonutrients, far more than green or white cabbage. Its rich, hearty flavour also makes a welcome change to carrots and broccoli. This is based on an old Jewish recipe and it goes very well with Sunday roast, grilled salmon or vegetarian sausages and mash.

1 tbsp olive oil or rapeseed oil
1 red onion
1 red cabbage
2 apples
75g dried apricots
4 tbsp red wine vinegar (about 60ml)
2 tbsp balsamic vinegar (about 30ml)
2 tbsp soft brown sugar
125ml stock

Preparation time: 15 minutes plus 1 hour simmering.
Equipment: 1 large pan.
Storage: Fridge for 24 hours or freeze.
Servings: 10–12.

- Peel and dice the red onion.
- Heat the oil in a pan and sauté the onion for 5 minutes.
- Meanwhile, cut the cabbage in half, lay it flat side down, cut in half again, then shred finely.
- Peel, core and dice the apples and roughly chop the apricots into pea-sized pieces.
- When the onion is ready, add all the other ingredients, mix, bring to the boil and then simmer for 1 hour with the lid on, stirring occasionally.

Butternut squash and goats' cheese parcels

Filo parcels with a delicious filling of creamy butternut squash and spinach combined with tangy goats' cheese. A great vegetarian alternative to a Sunday roast, or have them for lunch with a fresh leafy salad.

1 small onion
1 small butternut squash (about 200g peeled flesh)
1 tbsp rapeseed oil
2 cloves garlic
4 sage leaves
85g frozen spinach
60g soft goats' cheese
2 sheets frozen filo pastry

Preparation time: 25 minutes plus 12–15 minutes baking.
Equipment: 1 deep-sided frying pan with a lid and 1 baking tray.
Storage: Eat straightaway.
Servings: 2.

- Peel and dice the onion. Cut the peel off the butternut squash and dice into 1cm cubes. Finely chop the sage leaves.
- Heat 1 teaspoon of the oil in the frying pan and sauté the onion and crushed garlic for 2 minutes.
- Add the butternut squash, sage and 2 tablespoons of water, then cook with the lid on for 10 minutes, until tender. Add a little extra water if the mixture begins to stick to the bottom of the pan.
- Meanwhile, put the frozen spinach in a small bowl and microwave for 1 minute, then stir with a fork. Squeeze the spinach against the side of the bowl and drain away as much liquid as possible.

- Add the goats' cheese to the spinach.
- Preheat the oven to 180°C (160°C fan)/350°F/gas mark 4.
- When the butternut squash is ready, mix with the spinach and cheese and leave to cool slightly.
- Cut one sheet of filo pastry in half to make two squares. Brush one with some of the oil, then place on the baking tray, oiled side down. Place the second square on top of the first so that the corners don't match and you have an eight-cornered star. Brush a little more oil around the edges of the second square and place half the vegetable and cheese mixture in the centre. Pull up the edges of the pastry around the filling and pinch together to form a sack. Repeat to form a second parcel.
- Bake for 12–14 minutes, until golden brown.

Egg and watercress sandwich

If you think of egg sandwiches as something only pensioners eat, this will change your mind. Peppery watercress provides a great contrast to creamy egg and mayonnaise, and with some good granary bread you have the perfect sandwich.

2 slices granary, multigrain or seeded bread
1 egg
1 tbsp reduced fat mayonnaise
1 spring onion
1 large handful watercress
salt and pepper

Preparation time: 10–12 minutes.
Equipment: 1 small pan.
Storage: Fridge for 24 hours.
Servings: 1.

- Place the egg in a pan and cover with water to at least 1cm above it. Bring to the boil, and once you have large bubbles simmer for 8 minutes.
- Meanwhile, finely slice the spring onion and place in a bowl with the mayonnaise.
- There is no need for butter or margarine, but you can spread a little of the mayonnaise onto the top slice of bread.
- Prepare the watercress by removing any thick stems.
- When the egg is ready, immediately drain the water and replace it with cold water. Repeat a couple of times until the egg is cool enough to handle. If

you leave the egg in the boiling water, it will continue to cook and you'll get a dark line between the yolk and the white.

- Crack the egg against a hard surface and peel away the shell. Place the egg in the bowl and mash it with the other ingredients using a fork. Add a little salt and pepper to taste.
- Spread the egg over the bread, then top with watercress and the top slice of bread.

Tip

- If you're feeling hungry, have two eggs – they're good for keeping hunger at bay and much healthier than reaching for a biscuit.

Mayonnaise explained

While you're pregnant you shouldn't eat fresh mayonnaise, as it is made with raw eggs that could be contaminated with salmonella. However, it is fine to have mayonnaise such as Hellmann's or other brands from a supermarket, as these are made with pasteurised egg. You are only likely to come across fresh mayonnaise for sale if you go to a farm shop – you'll be able to spot that it's fresh as it will be stored in the fridge and have a short shelf life. Mayonnaise made with pasteurised eggs lasts for months. If you buy a sandwich or salad from a supermarket or high street shop, such as Greggs, Pret A Manger or Boots, any mayonnaise it contains will be made with pasteurised egg. If in doubt, maybe in an expensive restaurant or at a farmer's market or festival, just ask if the mayonnaise is home-made.

Creamy pea and tofu dip

This tastes light and delicious and is incredibly easy to make. Tofu is rich in calcium so will help you meet your extra requirements, and although you can't taste it in this dip it provides a lovely creamy texture.

100g frozen peas, defrosted
100g tofu
2 spring onions
2–3 mint leaves
1 tsp lemon juice
pinch cumin
1 clove garlic (optional)
salt and pepper

Preparation time: 5–10 minutes.
Equipment: 1 bowl or blender.
Storage: Fridge for 2 days or freeze.
Servings: 2–3.

- Drain the tofu and put it in the bowl, then add the peas.
- Roughly chop the spring onions and mint leaves into the bowl and, if you like garlic, add the crushed garlic too. Blend until smooth.
- Stir in the lemon juice and cumin and a little salt and pepper to taste.

Tip

- Serve with toasted pitta bread and vegetable sticks.

Cauliflower and chickpea curry

Curries tend to be very high in fat and calories but this is a healthy version that's packed with vegetables and still hits the spot.

1 tbsp olive oil
1 onion
1 clove garlic
1 tsp coriander
1 tsp cumin
1 tsp turmeric
½ red pepper
½ cauliflower
1 x 400g tin chickpeas
450ml stock
1 tbsp tomato puree
1 tbsp grated creamed coconut

Preparation time: 15 minutes plus 20 minutes simmering.
Equipment: 1 pan with a lid.
Storage: Fridge for 24 hours or freeze.
Servings: 2–3.

- Peel and dice the onion. Heat the oil in the pan and sauté the onion for 2–3 minutes.
- Stir in the crushed garlic and spices and cook for another minute.

- Remove the seeds from the pepper, wash and dice. Wash the cauliflower and cut into bite-sized pieces.
- Add the pepper, cauliflower, drained chickpeas, tomato puree and stock to the pan, bring to the boil and simmer with the lid on for 20 minutes, until the vegetables are tender.
- Stir in the creamed coconut and cook for a minute more to thicken.
- Serve with brown or basmati rice and some cucumber and mint raita (p123).

Tip

- If you especially like spicy food, add some chopped chilli at the same time as the spices.

> 66 *This was delicious. It was quick and easy to make and full of flavour.* 99
> **Victoria, 32 weeks pregnant**

Fact or fiction: Eating curry will bring on labour

This is a myth. However, if you have a curry that's so unbearably hot it causes stomach cramps and diarrhoea, it might also trigger contractions. The idea is that very spicy food stimulates the intestines in the same way as a dose of castor oil, causing spasms and moving everything rapidly through the bowels. If this happened, in theory it could also set off uterine contractions and bring on labour. However, if this were the case you'd be feeling decidedly the worse for wear, which isn't an ideal state for handling labour. So if your due date is a while off yet, don't worry that a mild curry will cause you to go into labour early. If you're overdue, enjoy your curry, but don't expect it to work miracles – babies come when they're ready.

Spinach dhal

This makes an easy supper with basmati rice and natural yogurt, or have it alongside your favourite chicken or vegetable curry. Leftovers go well with pasta or mixed with some stock to make a warming soup.

250g split yellow peas
700ml water
1 tbsp lemon juice
pinch of salt

1 tbsp olive oil or rapeseed oil
1 onion
3 cloves garlic
2 tsp grated fresh root ginger
1½ tsp ground cumin
1 tsp ground turmeric
½ tsp mild chilli powder
125g frozen spinach or 125g fresh spinach
black pepper

Preparation time: 20 minutes plus 50 minutes simmering.
Equipment: 1 pan and 1 frying pan.
Storage: Fridge for 24 hours or freeze.
Servings: 2 as a main course or 4 as a side dish.

- Rinse the split peas and add 700ml of water. Bring to the boil and simmer for about 50 minutes, stirring occasionally.
- Remove from the heat and stir in the lemon juice and salt, then set aside.
- Finely dice the onion.
- Heat the oil in the frying pan and fry the onion and crushed garlic for 5 minutes. Add the ginger and spices and cook for 2 minutes more.
- Add the spinach to the onion mixture and gently stir until heated through. If you're using fresh spinach, cook until nicely wilted.
- Stir the onion and spinach mixture into the split peas. Add black pepper and a little salt to taste.

Cucumber and mint raita

A cooling dressing to have with curry or other spicy food, or have it with salad, wraps or burgers.

125ml natural yogurt
¼ cucumber
2–4 mint leaves (according to taste)
1 tsp lemon juice
1 pinch cumin
1 pinch cayenne pepper

Preparation time: 10 minutes.
Pans: 1 bowl.

Storage: Fridge for 24 hours.
Servings: 2.

- Wash and finely grate the cucumber, then put it in the centre of a clean tea towel or a couple of sheets of strong kitchen paper. Draw together the corners and twist to squeeze out as much liquid as possible.
- Finely chop the mint leaves. If you start by rolling them up like a cigar it makes this easier.
- Mix all the ingredients together and serve with a couple of mint leaves on top.

Butternut squash and red lentil casserole

A delicious casserole to eat with a spoonful of natural yogurt on top and some basmati rice or couscous. It also freezes well, so you can enjoy it on a busy day in the future.

1 tbsp olive oil
1 onion
2 cloves garlic
2 tsp paprika
1 tsp ground cumin
1 tsp ground cinnamon
1 butternut squash
1 large sweet potato
1 red pepper
125g red lentils
1 x 400g tin chopped tomatoes
500ml stock

Preparation time: 20 minutes plus 30 minutes simmering.
Equipment: 1 casserole pan with a lid.
Storage: Fridge for 24 hours or freeze.
Servings: 4.

- Remove the skin and seeds from the butternut squash and dice. Peel and dice the sweet potato, and de-seed the pepper before dicing.
- Peel and dice the onion. Heat the oil in the pan and sauté the onion and crushed garlic for 5 minutes.
- Add the paprika, cumin and cinnamon to the pan, stir and cook for 2 minutes.

- Stir the vegetables into the onion mixture and cook for 1 minute.
- Add the lentils, tomatoes and stock, then bring to the boil and simmer for 30 minutes with the lid on, until the vegetables are tender. Stir occasionally while cooking.

Root vegetable rosti

Ideal for Sunday brunch or a leisurely lunch with scrambled egg and grilled tomatoes.

1 medium potato (about 200g peeled)
1 carrot (about 75g peeled)
1 parsnip (about 75g peeled)
2 spring onions
1 egg
salt and pepper
2 tsp olive oil or rapeseed oil

Preparation time: 25 minutes.
Equipment: 1 pan with a lid and 1 frying pan.
Storage: Fridge for 24 hours.
Servings: 2.

- Fill the kettle and turn on.
- Peel and coarsely grate the potato, carrot and parsnip into a pan.
- Cover with plenty of boiling water, bring back to the boil, then turn off the heat and leave for 5 minutes with the lid on.
- Finely chop the spring onions.
- Drain as much water as possible from the vegetables, then leave them to cool for a few minutes with the lid off.
- Turn the whole mixture out onto the centre of a clean tea towel. Pull together the corners into a bunch, then twist together to squeeze out as much water as possible.
- Return the vegetables to the pan and stir in the egg and spring onions.
- Heat one teaspoon of oil in the frying pan until sizzling hot, then pour in the vegetable mixture and turn the heat to medium. Spread the mixture out with a fish slice and press down.
- Cook for 4–5 minutes, then put a plate over the top of the pan and turn the pan upside down. Add another teaspoon of oil to the pan, then slide the rosti back in and cook the other side for 4–5 minutes.
- Turn out onto a clean plate and cut into wedges.

Rice and greens

This is packed with flavour as well as nutrients and makes a perfect accompaniment to grilled chicken or fish, or have it with chopped hard-boiled egg. Each portion provides two of your 5-a-day – and it includes kale, which is rich in calcium, iron and vitamins A, C and K.

1 small onion
2 tsp olive oil or rapeseed oil
1 clove garlic
100g brown basmati rice
450ml stock
100g kale
100g green beans (fresh or frozen)
100g frozen peas
freshly ground black pepper
1–2 tsp lemon juice

Preparation time: 30 minutes plus 25 minutes cooking.
Equipment: 1 pan.
Storage: Fridge 24 hours or freeze.
Servings: 2.

- Peel and dice the onion. Heat the oil in the pan and sauté with the crushed garlic for 2–3 minutes.
- Add the rice and stock, bring to the boil and simmer for 25 minutes with the lid on, until the rice is beginning to soften.
- Shred the kale and discard any tough pieces of stalk. Stir the kale into the rice and continue to cook.
- Top and tail the green beans if needed and chop into bite-sized pieces. Stir into the rice mixture and cook for about 10 minutes more, until tender.
- Stir the peas into the rice and cook for a few minutes, until completely heated through. Add a little extra water if the rice starts to stick to the bottom of the pan.
- Add lemon juice and black pepper to taste.

Tip

- Instead of kale you can use spring greens, cabbage or spinach. Asparagus can be substituted for green beans, and peas can be swapped for baby broad beans or soya beans.

66 *I'm trying to up my 5-a-day so this was ideal. I used spinach instead of kale and it was very tasty.* 99
Victoria, 32 weeks pregnant

Spicy fish tacos with avocado dressing

Fish tacos are popular in Mexico and the USA but are less well known here. The combination of warm, lightly spiced fish with a simple salad and creamy avocado, lime and coriander dressing makes a great lunch or light supper.

For the fish
2 fillets of white fish (e.g. river cobbler, cod, haddock)
2 tbsp plain white flour
½ tsp paprika
½ tsp ground cumin
½ tsp mild chilli powder
pinch salt
black pepper
2 tsp rapeseed oil

Avocado dressing
1 small avocado
75ml low fat natural yogurt
1 tbsp lime juice
1 tbsp fresh coriander

Salad
2 handfuls lettuce
2 tomatoes
¼ red onion
2 tbsp fresh coriander

To serve
2–4 soft corn or wheat tortillas

Preparation time: 25 minutes.
Equipment: 1 frying pan, 1 dinner plate, 1 small bowl and 1 salad bowl.
Storage: Eat straightaway.
Servings: 2.

- Start by preparing the salad: shred the lettuce, slice the tomatoes and thinly slice the red onion, then place in a bowl with the coriander leaves.
- To make the avocado dressing, chop the avocado in half, discard the stone and scoop out the flesh into a small bowl. Add the other ingredients and whiz with a hand-held blender until smooth.
- In the middle of a dinner plate, place the flour, paprika, cumin, chilli powder, salt and plenty of black pepper. If you like very spicy food, you can add a little more of the spices. Mix everything together.
- Cut the fish into strips about the size of a finger. Roll each one in the flour mixture and place at the edge of the plate.
- Heat the oil in the frying pan, then cook the fish strips for 4–5 minutes, turning occasionally.
- Meanwhile, place the tortillas directly on the shelves of an oven and turn to a medium heat – the temperature doesn't really matter, as you'll turn off the heat before it reaches that setting anyway. Remove from the oven when they're warm and you're ready to serve.
- To assemble each taco, place a warm tortilla on a plate, spread a few spoonfuls of dressing on it, scatter some salad over it, then add pieces of fish and a little more dressing. Roll up the taco and serve immediately. Any leftover salad can just be eaten on the side.

66 This hit the spot and felt like a really healthy dinner choice. I would never have thought of eating fish in a taco before and it has left me inspired to be more creative. I had it a second time around with chicken instead and that was also lovely. 99
Britt, 34 weeks pregnant

Mackerel and horseradish fishcakes

Mackerel is combined here with peppery horseradish for a fabulously flavoured fishcake that is coated with crispy breadcrumbs. These are a great way of including more oily fish in your diet.

250g unpeeled potatoes (e.g. Maris Piper)
2 mackerel fillets
2 spring onions
1 tbsp creamed horseradish
1 tbsp plain flour
1 egg
50g wholemeal breadcrumbs
2 tsp rapeseed oil

Preparation time: 45 minutes (and 30 minutes in the fridge if possible).
Equipment: 1 pan, 3 bowls or plates, 1 baking tray and 1 frying pan.
Storage: Fridge for 24 hours or freeze.
Servings: 2 (4 fishcakes).

- Peel the potatoes, cut them into chunks and put them in a pan. Cover with water and bring to the boil, then simmer for 10–15 minutes, until cooked.
- Cover your baking tray with foil, then place the mackerel fillets on the foil, skin side up. Place under a medium hot grill for 3–4 minutes, then turn over and grill for 3–4 minutes more.
- Cut the ends off the spring onions and chop finely.
- Beat the egg in a shallow bowl. Place the flour in another bowl or on a plate and the breadcrumbs in a third bowl or plate.
- When the fish is cooked, flake the fish off the skin using a fork. If you find any bones, remove them.
- Drain the potatoes and mash with a fork or potato masher, then stir in the fish, horseradish and spring onions.
- Take about a quarter of the mixture in your hands and form a fishcake shape. Place it on the floured plate to coat, then, with the fishcake on the flat palm of your hand, use a spoon or brush to cover it with egg. Turn it over to cover the other side. Next, sit the fishcake in the breadcrumbs and sprinkle the top and sides so that it is lightly coated. Place the fishcake on a plate. When you have four fishcakes, place them in the fridge for 30 minutes to firm up. If you don't have time for this, don't worry.
- Heat the oil in a frying pan and fry the fishcakes for 4–5 minutes on each side, until completely hot all the way through.

> 66 *These were extremely easy to make and were a success with our toddler and us alike.* 99
> **Corey, 34 weeks pregnant (and mum to Marcus, 18 months)**

Why you should eat oily fish

Oily fish, including salmon, mackerel and sardines, is rich in long-chain omega 3 fatty acids, especially DHA (docosahexaenoic acid). DHA is essential for the development of your baby's brain, nervous system and eyes, and although our bodies can make a small amount of DHA, pregnant women are advised to eat one or two portions of oily fish a week in order to meet their baby's needs. During this last trimester, your baby's brain is growing rapidly, so it's particularly important to have a good intake. As well as being important for pregnancy, DHA helps to keep your heart healthy and ward off dementia. Another reason your child might thank you for getting into the fish-eating habit!

Salmon and roast vegetables

Salmon with a honey and mustard marinade and roasted new potatoes and vegetables. Perfect for a hassle-free Sunday lunch but easy enough for a midweek supper.

350g baby new potatoes
2 salmon fillets or trout fillets
2 tsp olive oil
2 tsp honey
2 tsp wholegrain mustard
1 tbsp lemon juice
2 gloves garlic
100g fine green beans
1 red pepper
1 courgette

Preparation time: 20 minutes plus 25 minutes roasting.
Equipment: 1 roasting tin or shallow ovenproof dish, 1 pan and 1 bowl.
Storage: Fridge for 24 hours.
Servings: 2.

• Preheat the oven to 200°C (180°C fan)/400°F/gas mark 6. Brush some of the oil over the roasting tin.
• Put the new potatoes in a pan, cover with boiling water, bring back to the boil and simmer for about 20 minutes, until tender.
• In a bowl, combine the honey, mustard, lemon juice and the rest of the oil. Place the fish in the bowl to marinade and set aside.
• Slice the courgette into 1cm thick discs and chop the pepper into 2cm chunks.
• Remove the skins from the cloves of garlic and place the whole cloves in the roasting tin along with the courgettes, pepper and beans. Give the tin a gentle shake and place in the oven for 10 minutes.

- After 10 minutes, add the drained potatoes to the tin, place the salmon fillets of top and drizzle the remaining marinade over everything. If the fillets have skin on, place the fish skin side up.
- Place in the oven for 20–25 minutes, until the fish is cooked through and the vegetables are starting to brown.

Tips

- This also works well with baby sweetcorn, mange tout and cherry tomatoes.
- It tastes very nice served with reduced fat mayonnaise mixed with creamed horseradish on the side.

Grilled chicken burger with chunky guacamole

This makes you think of sunshine and health – super-tasty and packed with fresh flavours. Have it for lunch with some salad or for dinner with easy sweet potato wedges (p81).

2 chicken breasts

Marinade
½ lime, for juice
2 tsp rapeseed oil
2 tsp honey
½ tsp ground cumin

Chunky guacamole
1 avocado
1 tomato
2 tbsp finely diced red onion
½ lime, for juice
¼ tsp ground cumin
¼ tsp paprika
1 tsp fresh coriander or ¼ tsp ground coriander
¼ tsp finely diced red chilli (more if preferred)

To serve
2 granary rolls
4 tsp low fat mayonnaise

Preparation time: 30 minutes.
Pans: 1 baking tray and 1 bowl.
Storage: Eat straightaway.
Servings: 2.

- Place the chicken breasts between sheets of cling film and beat lightly using a mallet or rolling pin until about 1.5cm thick.
- Place the pieces of chicken on a baking tray covered with foil.
- In a small bowl, mix together the four ingredients for the marinade. Spread half the mixture on the top of the chicken breasts, then turn them over and spread the rest on the other side. Cover with cling film and place in the fridge for 10 minutes or longer.
- To prepare the guacamole, cut the avocado in half, discard the skin and stone and dice. Dice the tomato. Combine all the guacamole ingredients in a bowl and leave to stand at room temperature.
- When the chicken has marinated, place it under a medium hot grill for 6–7 minutes on each side, until it is slightly browned and the juices run clear.
- Meanwhile, cut the rolls in half and spread with mayonnaise.
- Place one piece of chicken on the bottom half of each roll and spoon the guacamole on top, followed by the top of the roll.

Chicken jalfrezi

A healthier version of this well-known chicken curry in tomato sauce. Great with rice or chapatti and natural yogurt.

1 tbsp rapeseed oil
1 onion
1 clove garlic
250g diced chicken breast
2 tsp ground turmeric
2 tsp ground cumin
½ tsp mild chilli or 1 red or green chilli (depending on taste)
1 x 400g tin chopped tomato
½ green pepper
1 tbsp grated fresh root ginger
2 tsp ground coriander
salt and pepper
2 tbsp fresh coriander
2–4 tbsp natural yogurt

Preparation time: 40 minutes.
Equipment: 1 deep-sided frying pan or casserole dish with a lid.
Storage: Fridge for 24 hours or freeze.
Servings: 2.

- Peel and dice the onion.
- Heat the oil in the pan and fry the onion with the crushed garlic for 2–3 minutes.
- Add the chicken, turmeric, cumin and chilli and fry for 5 minutes, turning the chicken so that all sides get cooked in the spices.
- Meanwhile, remove the stalk and seeds from the pepper and thinly slice.
- Add the pepper, tomatoes, grated ginger and ground coriander to the pan and stir well. Bring to the boil then simmer gently with the lid on for 10 minutes.
- Remove the lid and cook for 10 minutes more while the sauce reduces. Add salt and pepper to taste.
- Sprinkle chopped fresh coriander on top, then serve with a spoonful of yogurt.

Tip

- To make a vegetarian version, leave out the chicken and use mixed vegetables or add extra vegetables and paneer.

Fact or fiction: Your baby can taste your food

Your baby is not in there wrestling with a piece of toast, although it may feel that way, but she is getting familiar with flavour components from the foods you're eating. Believe it or not, the food you eat now will affect the taste preferences of your baby after birth. Research has shown that all babies are born liking sweet and salty flavours, but their preferences for many other flavours vary and are influenced by the foods the baby's mother eats during pregnancy. The amniotic fluid your baby is now swallowing contains substances from your diet that your baby can taste and smell. Studies have found that babies are more likely to enjoy garlic if their mothers ate it during pregnancy – likewise, it seems that eating a junk food diet during pregnancy could lead to similar preferences in your offspring. Some people believe that if your baby gets used to different vegetables, garlic and a wide range of other flavours during these months in the womb, you are less likely to be faced with a fussy eater when the time comes for weaning.

Spanish lamb stew

Lamb marinated with garlic, tomato and paprika, then slowly stewed with onion and green pepper. This involves very little hands-on time and makes a rich, warming stew that can be eaten with extra rice or potatoes and vegetables, depending on how hungry you're feeling.

▌ 250g lean lamb

▌ *Marinade*
1 clove garlic
1 bay leaf
75g tomato puree
½ tsp sugar
1 tbsp red wine vinegar
2 tbsp water

▌ 2 tsp olive oil
1 onion
1 green pepper
1 potato
250 ml water
1 tbsp fresh parsley or 1 tsp dried parsley
salt and freshly ground black pepper

Preparation time: 10 minutes plus 2 hours marinating, 15 minutes preparation and 1 hour simmering.
Equipment: 1 deep-sided frying pan or casserole pan with a lid and 1 mixing bowl.
Storage: Fridge for 24 hours or freeze.
Servings: 2.

- Trim any fat off the lamb and dice into bite-sized pieces.
- In a bowl, combine the crushed garlic with the other marinade ingredients and stir. Stir in the lamb to coat, then cover with cling film and place in the fridge for about 2 hours.
- Peel and dice the onion and remove the stalk and seeds from the pepper, then dice as well.
- Heat the oil in the pan and sauté the onion and pepper for 5 minutes, until soft.

- Meanwhile, peel and dice the potato.
- Add the potato, water, parsley and lamb to the pan along with any marinade remaining in the bowl. Bring to the boil, then simmer for about an hour, until the meat is tender.
- Add some pepper and a little salt if needed.

Tip

- This is another good one for doubling up – you can then put some in the freezer for the busier days to come.

Fact or fiction: When you cook alcohol it evaporates

This is true, but the amount of alcohol you're left with depends on how much you start with and how long you cook it for. When you heat a bottle of red wine for 5 minutes to make mulled wine, very little alcohol will evaporate, so you would still get one to two units of alcohol in a glass. The longer you cook a dish, the less alcohol remains: after 30 minutes, 35% of the alcohol is left; after an hour, only 25%; and after two and a half hours' cooking, just 5%. So, if you wanted to add wine to this stew, it would be absolutely fine. One portion of the stew would contain a grand total of 4% of a unit of alcohol, probably less than you'd get in one sip of wine.

Spiced pork with rice and green beans

A mildly spiced one-pot dish that's lovely and warming and takes very little preparation. Ideal if you're feeling tired and looking forward to putting your feet up.

250g diced pork (loin or topside)
2 tsp rapeseed oil
1 small onion
2 mushrooms
100g fine green beans
1 clove garlic
1 tsp ground cumin
1 tsp ground coriander
1 tsp paprika
¼ tsp cayenne pepper (if you like hotter food)
100g basmati rice
1 x 400g tin chopped tomatoes
250ml stock

Preparation time: 15 minutes plus 25 minutes simmering.
Pans: 1 deep-sided frying pan or wok with a lid.
Storage: Eat straightaway.
Servings: 2.

- Peel and dice the onion. Chop the mushrooms into wedges. Chop the ends off the beans and slice into 2.5cm pieces.
- Heat the oil in the frying pan and fry the onion for 3 minutes.
- Add the pork and fry for 2 minutes, until browned.
- Add the mushrooms, beans and garlic and cook for another minute.
- Stir in the spices, then the rice, and pour over the tin of tomatoes and the stock.
- Stir and bring to the boil, then simmer with the lid on for about 25 minutes, until the rice is cooked and the beans are tender.

Beef and cannellini bean hotpot

A simple, warming winter hotpot that can be eaten as it is or served with broccoli or green beans. Leftovers make a great lunch with crusty bread.

1 tbsp olive oil
1 onion
2 cloves garlic
400g lean minced beef
5 carrots
2 potatoes
2 sweet potatoes
1 bay leaf
2 tsp mixed herbs
1 tbsp Worcestershire sauce
550ml beef or vegetable stock
1 x 400g tin cannellini beans
2 tbsp tomato puree
2 tbsp cornflour

Preparation time: 20 minutes plus 30 minutes simmering.
Equipment: 1 casserole pan with a lid.
Storage: Fridge for 24 hours or freeze.
Servings: 4.

- Peel and dice the onion. Heat the oil in the pan and sauté the onion and crushed garlic for 5 minutes.
- Meanwhile, peel the carrots, potatoes and sweet potatoes. Chop the carrots into thick slices and the potatoes into bite-sized chunks.
- Add the minced beef to the onion and cook for about 5 minutes, stirring and breaking it up with a spoon until completely browned.
- Add the vegetables, bay leaf, herbs, Worcestershire sauce and stock and stir gently.
- Bring to the boil, then simmer with the lid on for 25–30 minutes, until the vegetables are tender.
- Mix the cornflour with 1–2 tablespoonfuls of cold water, then stir into the pan, along with the beans and tomato puree.
- Bring back to the boil and simmer for a few minutes before serving.

Desserts and snacks

Raspberry filo tarts

These look spectacular – delicate filo pastry shells with a creamy raspberry filling. Perfect for a dinner party or baby shower, and without the need for lots of cream and sugar.

1 sheet frozen filo pastry
2 tsp rapeseed oil
50q low fat cream cheese
50g low fat natural yogurt
1 tsp soft brown sugar
200g raspberries (fresh or frozen)
½ tsp icing sugar for dusting

Preparation time: 10 minutes plus 5 minutes baking.
Equipment: 1 muffin tray and 1 bowl.
Storage: Eat straightaway, or unfilled cases in an airtight container for a few days.
Servings: 4 tarts.

- Preheat the oven to 180°C (160°C fan)/350°F/gas mark 4.
- Using one teaspoon of oil, grease four holes in the muffin tray.
- Cut the sheet of filo pastry into eight squares.

- Brush oil over four of the squares, then press each one into a hole in the muffin tray, oiled side up. The corners will hang over the edges of the hole.
- Take each of the remaining squares and press them down gently on top of the squares in the tray. Instead of matching up the four corners, place the second sheet at an angle so the corners are mismatched.
- Bake for about 5 minutes, until the pastry is starting to brown. Leave to cool slightly before transferring to a cooling rack.
- In a bowl, mix the cream cheese, yogurt and brown sugar until smooth. Fold in about half the raspberries, then divide the mixture between the filo cases.
- Top with the remaining raspberries and dust with icing sugar.

Strawberries and cream trifle

Trifle is a great all-year-round pudding, often eaten at Christmastime but also in the summer. This recipe embraces trifle's best bits – fruity jelly, creamy custard and light whipped cream – but without the semi-cooked eggs and heavy creaminess. It looks pretty and you can make an indulgent version for special occasions or a low fat and low sugar type if preferred. Either way, it tastes delicious and provides you with a portion of fruit.

350g strawberries
1 pack strawberry jelly made up with 450ml water
6 sponge fingers
30g custard powder
15g sugar
300ml milk
60g squirty cream

Preparation time: 15 minutes plus setting time.
Equipment: 1 glass bowl.
Storage: Eat straightaway.
Servings: 4.

- Remove the stalks from the strawberries and slice half of them into the glass bowl. Break the sponge fingers into the bowl.
- Make the jelly by dissolving in 200ml of boiling water, then adding an additional 250ml. The instructions may say to use 580ml of water in total, but using slightly less makes for a stronger flavoured dish.
- Pour the jelly over the fruit and sponge, stir, and place in the fridge to set.

- Place the custard powder and sugar in a measuring jug and stir in enough of the milk to make a paste. Add the rest of the milk, mix, and place in the microwave for about 3 minutes, until thickened. Stir again, then leave to cool.
- Once the jelly, has set and the custard has cooled, you can stir the custard and pour it over the jelly, then leave it in the fridge until ready to eat.
- Just before serving, squirt cream over the top of the trifle and place the remaining strawberries on top.

Tips

- For a more indulgent pudding, you can use regular jelly, full fat milk and 200ml of whipping cream.
- For a lower-calorie version, use reduced sugar jelly, skimmed or semi-skimmed milk and half-fat squirty cream.
- Once the custard has cooled slightly, you can cover the jug with cling film to stop a skin forming on the top.
- You can replace the strawberries with fresh or frozen raspberries and scatter flaked almonds on top of the cream as well.

Fact or fiction: Fruit juices and smoothies are just as healthy as real fruit

It would make life easier if this were true, since having some orange juice with breakfast or grabbing a smoothie at lunch is so easy, but unfortunately it's not the case. Eating fruit in its natural state has several advantages. Firstly, it contains more fibre. When you eat an orange you got 20% of your day's fibre requirement, but have a glass of orange juice instead and you get virtually none. Secondly, pieces of fruit contain skin or pulp and therefore more cancer-fighting flavonoids. And finally, real fruit provides a slower release of sugar, which is particularly important during pregnancy. When you eat a piece of fruit, your digestive system has to work to break up the plant cell walls and release the nutrients, including the sugar. When you drink juice, this has already been done so the sugar is easily absorbed and quickly causes blood sugar levels to spike.

Sticky prune cake

A dark, sticky, very moist cake that's good for pudding with crème fraîche or ice cream, or mid-afternoon when energy levels are flagging.

1 tin of prunes (about 410g)
2 eggs
100ml rapeseed oil
125g plain flour
125g wholemeal flour
2 tsp baking powder
2 tsp mixed spice
1 tsp ground cinnamon
75g soft brown sugar
75g sultanas
1 tsp icing sugar for dusting

Preparation time: 15 minutes plus 35 minutes baking.
Equipment: 1 round cake tin (21cm or 24cm diameter) and 1 mixing bowl.
Storage: Airtight container for 2–3 days or freeze.
Servings: 10–12 slices.

- Preheat the oven to 180°C (160°C fan)/350°F/gas mark 4.
- Brush your cake tin with oil and line the bottom with greaseproof paper.
- Tip the whole tin of prunes, including the juice, into the mixing bowl. Squish each prune against the side of the bowl with a fork and remove the stone with your fingers.
- Crack the eggs into the bowl of prunes, add the oil and beat lightly with a fork.
- Add the flours, baking powder, mixed spice, cinnamon, sugar and sultanas and stir well.
- Transfer the mixture to your prepared cake tin and bake for 35–40 minutes.
- Leave the cake to cool in the tin for 5 minutes before turning out onto a cooling rack.
- Dust with icing sugar.

Chocolate brownie muffins

These are great when you need something chocolaty, but without lots of sugar and saturated fat. Avocados (yes avocados!) give the muffins a great texture as well as providing healthy monounsaturated fats, potassium, zinc and vitamins B6 and E.

2 ripe avocados
2 eggs
50ml rapeseed oil
100g caster sugar
100g plain flour
75g wholemeal flour
40g cocoa powder
2 tsp baking powder
1 tsp bicarbonate of soda
100ml milk
50g chopped walnuts

Preparation time: 15 minutes plus 12–15 minutes baking.
Equipment: 1 muffin tin and 1 mixing bowl.
Storage: Airtight container for a few days or freeze.
Servings: 12 muffins.

- Preheat the oven to 200°C (180°C fan)/400°F/gas mark 6. Place paper cake cases into the muffin tin.
- Cut the avocados in half, discard the stone and scoop out the flesh into a mixing bowl.
- Using a fork or a stick blender, mash or puree the avocado until smooth.
- Add the eggs, oil and sugar and whisk the mixture.
- Sift the cocoa powder, plain flour, baking powder and bicarbonate of soda into the bowl, then add the wholemeal flour and fold the dry ingredients gently in with the avocado mixture.
- Fold in the chopped walnuts and milk to make a smooth batter.
- Spoon the cake mixture into the cake cases and bake for 12–15 minutes, until well risen and spongy to the touch.

Fact or fiction: It's good to eat chocolate when you're pregnant

You'll be pleased to hear that this one is true – in moderation, of course. Scientists in Finland looked at stress levels and chocolate consumption among 200 pregnant women, then followed up how their babies were once they were six months old. Women who ate chocolate regularly throughout pregnancy were more likely to report that their baby was active and smiled and laughed a lot. Although chocolate is known to trigger the release of serotonin, the happy hormone, this is unlikely to be responsible for the results. It's probably the case that the women who had a bit of chocolate a few times a week felt good and more relaxed, which can only have a positive effect on their babies. Chocolate contains sugar and caffeine so you shouldn't have too much, but as an occasional treat it really does seem to do you good.

Carrot and Brazil nut cake

Everyone loves carrot cake but many recipes aren't as healthy as you might imagine. This one, however, is packed with nutritious ingredients. It contains selenium-rich Brazil nuts, which are great for men's health and also for pregnancy. It also contains dried apricots, which are a good source of iron, and they provide a lovely tangy flavour to balance the Brazils.

225g carrots
75g Brazil nuts
75g dried apricots
125ml rapeseed oil
3 eggs
100g soft brown sugar
100g wholemeal flour
125g plain flour
2 tsp baking powder
½ tsp bicarbonate of soda
1½ tsp ground mixed spice

Icing
100g reduced fat cream cheese
50g icing sugar
½ tsp vanilla essence

Preparation time: 25 minutes plus 45 minutes baking.
Equipment: 1 mixing bowl and 1 round cake tin (20cm to 25cm diameter).
Storage: Airtight container for 2–3 days or freeze. Once iced it should be stored in the fridge.
Servings: 1 large cake.

- Preheat the oven to 180°C (160°C fan)/350°F/gas mark 4. Grease the cake tin using some of the oil and line the bottom with greaseproof paper.
- Peel and finely grate the carrots into the mixing bowl.

- Chop the Brazil nuts and apricots as finely as you like. They should be pea-sized or much smaller if you prefer. Add to the carrots.
- Pour the oil into a measuring jug, then add the eggs and beat well. Add to the mixing bowl along with the sugar and stir well.
- Add the flours, baking powder, bicarbonate of soda and mixed spice and gently combine all the ingredients.
- Transfer the mixture to the cake tin and smooth out. Bake for 40–45 minutes, until a skewer inserted in the centre comes out dry.
- Leave to cool in the tin for 5–10 minutes before moving to a cooling rack.
- When the cake has cooled, mix together the ingredients for the icing and smooth over the top of the cake.

Why you should eat selenium-rich foods

Selenium is a powerful antioxidant nutrient that is found in high quantities in Brazil nuts. It's often talked about for its role in protecting men from prostate cancer, but it is also important for you and your baby. Research suggests that it may offer protection against raised blood pressure, pre-eclampsia and premature labour. Selenium is also vital for a healthy immune system, and research suggests that having a good intake during pregnancy may help protect babies from developing eczema and wheezing in the first few years of life. While Brazil nuts are by far the richest source of selenium, you can also find it in tuna, white fish such as cod, lentils and bread.

Chocolate popcorn

Popcorn is one of the healthiest snacks around. It's a whole grain and so provides fibre and minerals and helps keep hunger at bay. If you cover it in butter, salt and caramel, it's obviously not so healthy, but there are plenty of other ingredients you can add that are much better for you. A portion of this delicious chocolate popcorn provides 200 calories.

50g popping corn
20g dark chocolate
oil for greasing if your pan isn't non-stick

Preparation time: 5 minutes.
Equipment: 1 pan with a lid.
Storage: Eat straightaway.
Servings: 2.

- Brush the base of the pan with a little oil if it isn't non-stick.
- Put the popcorn kernels into the pan, put the lid on and place on a high heat.
- Finely grate the chocolate while you wait for the corn to start popping.
- When you hear the first pop, give the pan a shake, making sure you hold onto the pan handle with one hand and the lid with the other.
- Lift the pan and give it another quick shake every so often until the popping stops, then turn off the heat and count to at least 10 before removing the lid.
- Pour the hot popcorn into a bowl, sprinkle the chocolate on top and stir with a spoon so the chocolate coats the corn as it melts.

Tips

- To make cheesy popcorn, add 15g of Cheddar or Parmesan cheese and ¼ teaspoon of paprika to the warm corn.
- To make honey nut corn, add a tablespoon of warmed honey and 2 tablespoons of finely chopped nuts.

Gruyère and green olive oaties

These are like savoury flapjacks with the nutty taste of Gruyère cheese. If you're avoiding big meals before bed, these make a good snack in the evening, as the oats provide slow-release energy.

2 eggs
200g oats
2 tbsp rapeseed oil
50g Gruyère cheese
50g mature Cheddar
50g pitted green olives

Preparation time: 10 minutes plus 20 minutes baking.
Equipment: 1 baking tray (20cm x 30cm) and 1 mixing bowl.
Storage: Airtight container for a few days or freeze.
Servings: 18 biscuits.

- Preheat the oven to 180°C (160°C fan)/350°F/gas mark 4. Cover the baking tray with a sheet of greaseproof paper.
- Crack the eggs into the mixing bowl and beat lightly.
- Add the oats, oil, grated cheese and roughly chopped olives. Mix well.

- Transfer the mixture to the baking tray and spread out.
- Bake for 20 minutes, until the edges are starting to brown slightly.
- Mark into slices, then leave to cool for 5 minutes before transferring to a cooling rack.

Drinks

Mildly spiced bedtime milk

If heartburn, restless legs or your growing bump are keeping you awake at night, this will have you sleeping like a baby. Well, it should help at least. Cardamom and ginger are traditionally thought to aid digestion and warm milk and nutmeg are reputed to help with sleep.

1 cup milk
1 heaped tsp grated fresh root ginger
2 cardamom pods
pinch nutmeg

Preparation time: 8 minutes.
Equipment: 1 small jug.
Storage: Drink straightaway.
Servings: 1.

- Peel the ginger and grate into the jug.
- Crush the cardamom pods and add the pods and seeds to the jug.
- Add a pinch of nutmeg and the milk, then microwave for about 2 minutes, until steaming hot but not boiling.
- Leave for 5 minutes, then pour through a tea strainer into a clean mug.

How to treat heartburn

Heartburn is fairly common in pregnancy, as the muscle valve that usually prevents the acidic stomach contents from going back up the food pipe becomes more relaxed. In the third trimester, it can become particularly bad as your stomach also becomes squashed by your growing baby. You may be able to help prevent it by having smaller portions and less fluid at mealtimes, so you don't become too full. Also try sitting up straight when you eat and for a while afterwards. Some women find citrus fruits or tomatoes can be a trigger, while others say bananas or tea make things worse. Alternative therapies, including aromatherapy and yoga, can ease the problem considerably for some, but if you suffer from severe heartburn, it's best to talk to your midwife or doctor about getting a suitable medicine.

Third trimester meal planner

Although following a meal plan isn't necessary, this schedule shows what a healthy diet looks like for the third trimester. As well as plenty of fruit, vegetables and starchy carbohydrate-rich foods, it includes more snacks to supply the extra nutrients you need at this stage. Eating smaller meals and more snacks may also help you to feel more comfortable. The planner also includes lots of different flavours to help your baby become familiar with different tastes.

This meal plan meets the requirements for energy, protein, potassium, calcium, magnesium, phosphorus, iron, copper, zinc, chloride, selenium, iodine, thiamin, riboflavin, niacin and vitamins A, B6, B12, C and E.

To meet all the nutrient requirements for this stage of pregnancy, you would also need to take a supplement containing 10μg vitamin D (see p9) and have plenty of water or other drinks.

Day 1

Breakfast: Breakfast bruschetta (p107)
Lunch: Italian fish soup (p111), garlic bread
Dinner: Butternut squash and red lentil casserole (p124), couscous, yogurt, sticky prune cake (p139) and half-fat crème fraîche
Snacks: Banana, slice of toast with reduced fat cream cheese, chocolate Brazil nuts

Day 2

Breakfast: Branflakes with milk and sliced banana
Lunch: Egg and watercress sandwich (p119), an apple, a glass of orange juice
Dinner: Beef and cannellini bean hotpot (p136), broccoli, a slice of cheesecake
Snacks: Slice of granary toast with honey, dried apricots, mildly spiced bedtime milk (p145)

Day 3

Breakfast: Apple, prune and almond bircher muesli (p109)
Lunch: Cheese and tomato toasted wholemeal sandwich
Dinner: Mackerel and horseradish fishcakes (p128), mixed salad
Snacks: Fruit yogurt, a banana, sticky prune cake (p139)

Day 4

Breakfast: Apple, prune and almond bircher muesli (p109) with sliced strawberries
Lunch: Tuna mayonnaise and sweetcorn sandwich, a small packet of crisps
Dinner: Roast chicken, roast potatoes, braised red cabbage (p117), peas and carrots, gravy, strawberries and cream trifle (p138)
Snacks: Pear, a handful of mixed nuts and raisins, mildly spiced bedtime milk (p145)

Day 5

Breakfast: Weetabix and sliced banana
Lunch: Chicken, reduced fat mayonnaise and salad sandwich, grapes
Dinner: Cauliflower and chickpea curry (p121), brown basmati rice, cucumber and mint raita (p123)
Snacks: Chocolate popcorn (p143), a small croissant, a small bowl of muesli

Day 6

Breakfast: Muesli, a glass of orange juice
Lunch: Root vegetable rosti (p125), scrambled egg, baked beans
Dinner: Grilled chicken burger with chunky guacamole (p131), baked potato and sliced tomatoes
Snacks: Carrot and Brazil nut cake (p142), plums, yogurt

Day 7

Breakfast: Carrot cake porridge (p163)
Lunch: Mediterranean couscous salad (p113), houmous, carrot sticks
Dinner: Spaghetti bolognaise, raspberry filo tart (p137)
Snacks: Oatcakes with Cheddar, grapes, chocolate popcorn (p143)

5 Breastfeeding

The early days of life with a new baby go by in something of a blur, especially if you're trying to establish breastfeeding as well as get some sleep. Your body has been through a lot, so, as well as resting and sleeping, it's important to eat well and drink plenty of fluids to aid your recovery and help your milk supply.

Try to eat regular meals throughout the day. You may not be a breakfast person, but if you've been breastfeeding in the night and you're going to be feeding in the day, you need the fuel. Lunch is also important, as you want your baby to get as much milk as possible during the daytime so she will hopefully sleep at night. You're probably used to having your biggest meal in the evening, but eating a good breakfast and lunch is now more important. Try to base the meals around starchy carbohydrates and have cereal or toast for breakfast, or both. Eggs are also a quick and nutritious food for the morning and there are a couple of recipes in this section to inspire you (pp152 and 153). At lunchtime have a sandwich with thick granary bread or maybe a big baked potato or pasta salad. If you find you're busy breastfeeding at lunchtime, then make a sandwich earlier in the day and put it in the fridge, so it's ready when you want it. Babies often enjoy a morning nap and this is a good time to make yourself something for later. Soup is another option, as you can heat it up at lunchtime and just grab some bread to go with it (pp155 and 156).

A healthy diet for breastfeeding includes:

- at least five portions of fruit and vegetables every day – try to vary these as much as possible
- protein foods, such as meat, fish, eggs, milk, beans and pulses
- starchy carbohydrate-rich foods including rice, pasta, bread and breakfast cereal – get your extra calories from these rather than from biscuits or other sugary snacks

- high-fibre foods such as vegetables, pulses and wholemeal bread and pasta – these will supply extra vitamins and minerals and help prevent constipation, which can be a particular problem in the early days
- high-calcium foods, especially milk, yogurt and cheese, to meet your extra requirements (p154)
- iron-rich foods including meat, fish, breakfast cereals and pulses (p110) – these will help replenish your iron stores
- zinc-rich foods to meet your increased requirements in pregnancy (p174), for example meat, poultry, milk and wholegrain cereal products
- oily fish such as salmon and sardines to supply long-chain omega 3 fatty acids and increase your baby's intake of these healthy fats.

Losing weight and getting back into pre-pregnancy clothes is an issue for many women, but it's not something to rush. At this stage it is better to focus on staying healthy and producing plenty of breast milk for your baby. It is estimated that breastfeeding uses up about 500 calories a day, but this varies according to how much milk your baby is taking. If you're feeding a 5-month-old baby who's not having anything else to eat or drink, you'll obviously produce more milk than someone who's feeding a 1-month-old baby and giving top-up bottles. The best indicator of how many calories you need a day is your weight. It's not a good idea to lose weight too quickly, but if you need to shed the pounds, don't make the mistake of thinking it will happen automatically just because you're breastfeeding (see p178).

Breastfeeding is surprisingly thirsty work, and drinking is just as important as eating well. Every time you sit down with your baby, make sure you have a big glass of water by your side. Even if you don't feel thirsty when you start, you might find you're gasping for a drink after a few minutes' feeding. Don't force yourself to drink if you don't feel like it, but keep well hydrated. This will make it easier for your body to produce breast milk and help you avoid getting headaches. Drinks made with milk or yogurt are particularly good, as they provide some of the extra calcium you need – you can whiz some up with fruit to make a shake, or look at the recipes on pp154 and 180 for inspiration.

When you're breastfeeding, you no longer need to avoid the long list of cheeses and other foods that were off limits during pregnancy. If you've been dreaming of runny eggs or a nice piece of Camembert, you can now feel free to enjoy them. You should still be careful about food hygiene and 'use by' dates, but you're no more likely than other adults to get food poisoning. Although there are no foods you need to completely avoid while breastfeeding, there are some you need to limit.

- Don't eat more than one portion of swordfish, marlin or shark per week.
- Don't eat more than two portions of oily fish per week, e.g. salmon, mackerel or fresh tuna (tinned tuna is fine while breastfeeding).
- Try not to have too much caffeine. There's no official limit but sticking to the 200mg per day limit for pregnancy is sensible (p8).
- As a general rule, have no more than one or two units of alcohol once or twice a week.

Supplements

The government advises women to take 10μg of vitamin D per day while they are breastfeeding. This is because many women have been found to have low levels in their blood, which means their baby receives less vitamin D from the breast milk they produce. It's important your baby has a good intake, as it helps with calcium absorption and the formation of strong, healthy bones.

If you were anaemic during pregnancy or lost a significant amount of blood when your baby was born, then an iron supplement may also be a good idea. You might be given a blood test to check your iron levels but this doesn't always happen.

If you're having trouble establishing breastfeeding, then the importance of eating well, drinking plenty and resting can't be overemphasised. Good positioning is key, of course, and if you're having any problems with feeding, keep asking for help. Midwives, health visitors, the NCT and the National Breastfeeding Helpline should all be able to offer advice. There is no such thing as poor-quality milk, but it can take time in the early days to get breastfeeding established. You may be used to being capable and efficient but now is the time to let other people help out. Let someone else make the dinner – many of the recipes here are simple enough for complete novices – and leave them to wash up too. And if your house is messier than you'd like, try not to worry – it's more important to look after yourself right now.

Breakfasts

Toasted coconut muesli with raspberries

A nutty, oaty breakfast with fresh raspberries and natural yogurt. It's low in sugar and high in fibre and antioxidants.

80g oats
25g desiccated coconut
15g flaked almonds
2 tsp honey
1 tbsp water
175g raspberries
200g low fat natural yogurt

Preparation time: 5 minutes plus 20 minutes baking.
Equipment: 1 bowl and 1 baking tray.
Storage: Airtight container for 1–2 weeks.
Servings: 2.

- Preheat the oven to 130°C (110°C fan)/250°F/gas mark ½.
- In a bowl, mix together the oats, coconut, almonds, honey and water.
- Spread out on a baking tray and bake for 20 minutes, until golden brown.
- Leave to cool completely before storing in an airtight container.
- Serve with a little milk and place the yoghurt and raspberries on top.

Tips

- You can substitute bananas or other fruit for the raspberries.
- It's very easy to make more portions at the same time but make sure you use extra baking trays so that the mixture is in just a thin layer.

Why you shouldn't use espressos to stay awake

There is no official limit to the amount of caffeine you can drink while you're breastfeeding, but it is known that caffeine passes into breast milk, so while you enjoy a morning cuppa so does your baby. There's no evidence to suggest that a mug of tea will do any harm, but it's not a good idea to start the day with a double espresso, even if you feel like one after a sleepless night. We don't really know how caffeine affects babies, and while some experts say it doesn't seem to do them any harm, others believe it can make babies unsettled and irritable. The truth is probably that some babies, like some adults, are more sensitive to the effects of caffeine than others. It's certainly worth keeping an eye on your baby to see if you notice any links between her behaviour and your caffeine intake. Babies aren't as good at metabolising caffeine as adults, so it can stay in their system for longer. This seems to be particularly true for younger babies. Another issue is that drinking lots of tea and coffee can lead to dehydration, so every time you have a cup of tea or coffee, try to match it with a glass of water to keep your fluid levels up

Mexican breakfast burrito

Egg, avocado and sliced tomato make a healthy breakfast or brunch combination, especially if you have them in a seeded wrap. You can have this as it is, spice it up with chillies or add coriander, depending on how you're feeling.

1 wrap (wholemeal or seeded if possible)
½ ripe avocado
1 tomato
1 egg
salt and freshly ground black pepper
½ tsp rapeseed oil
2 tsp tomato puree or ketchup
squeeze of lime juice
1 spring onion (optional)
1 tbsp fresh coriander (optional)
¼ tsp diced red chilli (optional)

Preparation time: 5–10 minutes.
Equipment: 1 small frying pan.
Storage: Eat straightaway.
Servings: 1.

- Beat the egg in a small cup or bowl with a little salt and pepper.
- Slice the avocado and tomato and finely chop the spring onion, coriander and chilli, if using.
- Place the wrap in the oven and turn it on at a medium heat to warm through. The temperature doesn't matter, as you'll turn the oven off in a few minutes.
- Heat the oil in the frying pan and pour in the egg. Leave for a minute, then break it up and turn over. When the egg is set, turn off the heat.
- Place the wrap on a warm plate, spread the tomato puree over it, then arrange the slices of tomato and avocado in a line down the centre, along with any other additions.
- Squeeze some lime juice over the filling, then place the egg on top, roll up the wrap and cut it in half.

Tomato poached eggs

After nine months of not being able to have runny yolks, this dish is bliss – a perfect pairing of rich tomato sauce and eggs with golden yellow yolks! It makes an easy breakfast, brunch or lunch with lightly toasted crusty bread.

1 x 400g tin chopped tomatoes
2 tsp olive oil
2 cloves garlic
1 tbsp tomato puree
1 tsp sweet paprika or regular paprika
½ tsp dried parsley or 2 tsp fresh parsley
¼ tsp sugar
salt and pepper
4 eggs

To serve
bread

Preparation time: 20 minutes.
Equipment: 1 frying pan or an iron skillet with a lid or a baking tray to lay on top.
Storage: Eat straightaway.
Servings: 2.

- Heat all the ingredients, apart from the eggs, in the pan. Simmer for 8–10 minutes, until reduced slightly.
- Break the eggs into the sauce as far apart as possible so that each one is surrounded by sauce. Add a little more black pepper. Cover and simmer over a medium low heat for 5 minutes, until the egg whites are set and the yolks are still runny.
- Serve on top of warm toast or in the pan, with more salt and pepper if needed and bread for dipping.

Tips

- You can make a Middle Eastern version of this dish, called shakshuka, by frying some onions and peppers in the pan before adding the tomato, and seasoning with cumin, coriander, thyme, parsley and saffron.
- A Mexican version, huevos rancheros, is also delicious. It has thinly sliced chillies added and is served on top of a warm tortilla or wrap to soak up the juices.

- You can also make your own variation by cooking onions, shallots, peppers, courgettes or mushrooms before adding the chopped tomatoes.

Why you should eat eggs

Eggs are the ultimate convenience food for busy new mums. They contain protein and almost all the essential vitamins and minerals. Two eggs will provide half of your daily vitamin D requirements and one-third of your iodine, which many new mums miss out on. If you don't get enough of these nutrients in what you eat, then your baby won't get enough from your breast milk, so it's important to include them in your diet. Both vitamin D and iodine are often in short supply, because they're found in only a small number of foods, including fish, eggs and milk. So make the most of eggs with easy dishes like scrambled eggs, omelettes, frittatas and Spanish tortillas.

Strawberry and yogurt smoothie

Start the day with a refreshing calcium-boosting smoothie. Have it with toast and peanut butter or your favourite spread for a really nutritious breakfast.

5 medium strawberries
½ banana
100g low fat natural yogurt
50ml milk

Preparation time: 5 minutes.
Equipment: 1 blender.
Storage: Fridge for 24 hours.
Servings: 1.

- Wash the strawberries and remove the stalks.
- Place everything in the blender and blend until smooth.

Why you should eat more calcium-rich foods.

When you were pregnant your body needed about 700mg of calcium a day. Now you're breastfeeding your requirement increases to 1,250mg. That's equivalent to more than a pint and a half of milk every single day. If you don't get enough calcium, it probably won't be your baby who suffers. Your breast milk will still contain all the calcium she needs, but you could be risking your own bone health for the future. The easiest way to increase your calcium intake is to have more milk, yogurt and cheese. But remember to choose low fat versions such as skimmed or semi-skimmed milk, low fat yogurt and reduced fat cheeses. Calcium is also found in tofu, almonds, curly kale and tinned sardines (since you eat the bones too). However, if you don't eat dairy products, you're unlikely to get enough calcium just from these alternatives, so you should look for a soya milk with added calcium or take a supplement.

Lunches, dinners and sides

Sweet potato and butter bean soup

A Moroccan-inspired soup that's easy to prepare and made with sweet potatoes and beans for slow energy release.

1 tbsp olive oil
1 red onion
1 clove garlic
1 large sweet potato
1 tsp ground cumin
1 tsp ground coriander
½ tsp cinnamon
½ tsp paprika
1 x 400g tin butter beans
500ml stock
salt and pepper
1 tbsp natural yogurt (optional)

Preparation time: 15 minutes plus 15–20 minutes simmering.
Equipment: 1 pan.
Storage: Fridge for 24 hours or freeze.
Servings: 4.

- Peel the onion, cut it in half, and then slice thinly. Heat the oil in the pan, then add the onion and crushed garlic and sweat, without browning, over a low heat for 2–3 minutes with the lid on.
- Meanwhile peel the sweet potato and cut into 1–2cm chunks.
- Add the spices to the onion and cook for a minute while stirring.

- Add the sweet potato, butter beans and stock. Bring to a gentle boil, then simmer with the lid on for 15–20 minutes, until the potato is tender.
- This soup tastes best with lots of whole beans and chunks of potato – if you use a stick blender, give it just a couple of 1 or 2 second pulses to thicken it up beautifully.
- Add salt and pepper to taste and serve with a spoonful of yogurt on top.

Corn chowder

A creamy, warming soup made with sweetcorn, which provides wholegrain carbohydrates, protein and fibre as well as a host of micronutrients, including vitamin C, B vitamins and potassium.

1 tbsp rapeseed oil or olive oil
1 onion
1 clove garlic
1 large potato
200g sweetcorn (fresh, frozen or tinned)
1 bay leaf
¼ tsp cayenne pepper
500ml stock
100ml milk

To serve
fresh parsley (optional)
salt and pepper to taste

Preparation time: 15 minutes plus 15 minutes cooking.
Equipment: 1 pan.
Storage: Fridge for 24 hours or freeze.
Servings: 4.

- Peel and dice the onion.
- Heat the oil in the pan and sweat the onion and crushed garlic for 3–4 minutes with the lid on.
- Meanwhile, peel the potato and chop into 2cm chunks.
- Add about half the corn to the pan along with the potato, bay leaf, cayenne pepper and stock. Bring to the boil, then simmer for about 10 minutes, until the potato is tender.
- Remove the bay leaf and roughly puree the soup with a hand-held blender.

- Add the milk and remaining corn and simmer for about 5 minutes.
- Season to taste and sprinkle the chopped parsley on top, if using.

Fact or fiction: If you eat a healthy diet your breast milk will be more nutritious

This is true. Some nutrients, including carbohydrates and protein, seem to be the same in all breast milk, but the amount of different fatty acids it contains varies depending on how much the mother eats. Women who eat more butter have been found to have more saturated fat in their milk and those who eat oily fish produce milk with higher levels of the beneficial long-chain omega 3 fatty acids. Vitamin B12 is another important nutrient that your baby will miss out on if you have a low intake yourself. Most people get more than enough of the vitamin if they eat a varied diet, including meat, fish, eggs and dairy foods, but vegans and women eating very little animal produce can miss out. In fact, there have been cases where breastfed babies have become deficient in vitamin B12, so if you eat a vegan or near-vegan diet it's important to take a B12 supplement. Vitamin D levels in breast milk also vary with intake. As many women have a poor diet, it is recommended that you take a supplement containing 10µg of vitamin D as a precaution.

Tabbouleh

A Middle Eastern salad made with bulgur wheat and fresh parsley and mint. Good with meatballs, kebabs and falafel or with houmous, salad and wraps.

75g bulgur
300ml water
40g chopped fresh parsley
10g fresh mint
2 spring onions
2 tbsp lemon juice
1 tbsp olive oil
1 clove garlic
½ tsp ground coriander
½ tsp ground cumin
¼ tsp mixed spice
2 tomatoes
5cm cucumber
salt and freshly ground black pepper

Preparation time: 25 minutes.
Equipment: 1 pan and 1 mixing bowl.
Storage: Fridge for 24 hours.
Servings: 2 as a main meal or 4–6 as a side dish.

- Place the bulgur in a pan with the water. Bring to the boil, then simmer for about 15 minutes with the lid on, until the water has been absorbed.
- Meanwhile, remove any tough stalks from the parsley (thin stems are fine) and remove the stems from the mint leaves. Finely chop the parsley, mint and spring onions with a sharp chopping knife – using a food processor tends to produce a mush. Place these in the mixing bowl.
- When the bulgur is cooked, stir in the lemon juice, olive oil, crushed garlic, coriander, cumin and mixed spice and leave to cool with the lid off.
- Dice the tomatoes and cucumber into pieces no larger than 1cm.
- Add the bulgur, tomatoes and cucumber to the mixing bowl and stir well to combine all the ingredients.
- Add salt and pepper to taste and more lemon juice if wanted.

Tips

- Instead of bulgur wheat, you can make this with couscous or quinoa.
- The weight of herbs given is for the amount you will actually use once the thick stems have been discarded, so you will need to buy packs weighing more than this.

Quick and simple curly kale

Kale is delicious and nutritious and is growing in popularity, not just among green juice health evangelists but even among those who might turn up their noses at cabbage and spinach. It has lots to offer, including more than twice as much iron, calcium and vitamins A and C as cabbage. If you've never eaten it before you might be pleasantly surprised, especially if you try this easy recipe to really bring out its best.

200g bag shredded kale
1 tsp olive oil or rapeseed oil
1 clove garlic
½ small onion
150ml boiling stock or water
2 tbsp red wine vinegar

Preparation time: 8 minutes.
Equipment: 1 deep-sided frying pan.
Storage: Fridge for 24 hours.
Servings: 2–3.

- Peel and very finely dice the onion.
- Heat the oil in the frying pan and sauté the onion with the crushed garlic for 1–2 minutes.
- Add the kale to the pan, removing any very thick woody stems, and stir in the stock. Cover and cook for 5 minutes over a medium hot heat.
- Add the vinegar, heat through, then serve.

Fact or fiction: Eating foods such as cabbage and onions will give your baby colic

Tiny components of the food you eat pass into your breast milk, and some women find that when they have particular foods their baby becomes more unsettled. However, most cases of colic are not related to the mother's diet, and the majority of babies don't suffer any problems when their mothers eat cabbage or any other food. If you suspect something you're eating is affecting your baby's behaviour, keep a diary to see if you can identify any pattern. Other foods that occasionally cause problems include tea and coffee, alcohol, wheat, fish, chocolate and citrus fruit or orange juice. Before cutting anything out of your diet, it's a good idea to talk to your doctor, midwife or health visitor to make sure you're not cutting out foods unnecessarily and that you're not missing out on essential nutrients.

Portobello mushroom burger

A super-simple vegetarian recipe that non-vegetarians will love as well. A whole cooked Portobello mushroom topped with houmous and feta in a granary roll – it provides plenty of flavour and all the important food groups in one go.

1 Portobello mushroom
pinch paprika
pinch mixed herbs
granary roll
1 heaped tbsp reduced fat houmous
1 tomato

handful lettuce
20g feta cheese

Preparation time: 5 minutes.
Equipment: 1 plate.
Storage: Eat straightaway.
Servings: 1.

- Place the mushroom on a microwave-safe plate, smooth side down, and sprinkle with the paprika and herbs. Cover and place in the microwave for about 4 minutes, until cooked but not soggy.
- Meanwhile, cut the roll in half and spread both sides with houmous. Slice the tomato and place on the bottom half and prepare the lettuce and feta.
- Place the cooked mushroom on the base of the roll. Crumble the feta on top, followed by the lettuce and the lid of the roll.

Baked tofu

Tofu is low in fat and rich in calcium so it's ideal when you're breastfeeding. It doesn't have a great reputation, however, as it's often cooked badly. The secret to making delicious tofu, rather than spongy tasteless tofu, is marinating it and drying it out well. This involves several steps but is actually very easy and doesn't require much hands-on time. Once the tofu is baked, you can use it to make healthy and delicious salads, stir-fries and wraps.

1 pack tofu (about 350g)
1 tbsp soya sauce
1 tbsp rice vinegar or white wine vinegar
1 tsp sesame oil

Preparation time: 5 minutes plus 15 minutes draining, at least 30 minutes marinating and 30 minutes baking.
Equipment: 1 bowl and 1 baking tray.
Storage: Fridge for 1–2 days or freeze.
Servings: 2–3.

- Drain the liquid from the tofu.
- Take two clean tea towels and fold them to about the size of the tofu block. Place one on a plate and put the tofu on top. Then place the second one on top of the tofu and put a chopping board on top. Now put something

heavy on top, such as a casserole dish, a heavy pan, or tins of beans. Leave for 15 minutes.

- Prepare the marinade by mixing together the soya sauce, vinegar and sesame oil in a bowl or airtight container.
- Slice the tofu into approximately 2cm cubes or small batons, then place in the bowl and gently coat with the marinade, either by turning the container upside down or with a spoon. Place in the fridge for at least 30 minutes – you can leave it overnight if that's easier.
- Preheat the oven to 200°C (180°C fan)/400°F/gas mark 6. Place a piece of greaseproof paper on the baking tray or brush it with a little oil.
- Arrange the tofu pieces in a single layer on the baking tray. Bake for 30 minutes, turning halfway through.
- The pieces can now be left aside to cool, ready for adding to your salad or stir-fry – or even for just eating on their own.

Tips

- You can use kitchen paper instead of tea towels, but a surprisingly large amount of liquid comes out of the tofu so you'll need quite a lot.
- You can add other ingredients to the marinade to give it extra flavour, depending on what you're going to use the tofu for, for example crushed garlic, grated ginger or chilli flakes.

Baked tofu salad

Once you've baked your tofu using the recipe above, you can use it to make this simple but flavour-packed salad. Tastes good with a wrap spread with houmous or with crusty bread – or, if you have any leftover brown rice or pasta, mix that in.

1 pack tofu – baked as described on p160
3 spring onions
2 carrots
2 tomatoes
1 small avocado
2 handfuls baby spinach or other salad leaves
50g frozen soya beans, peas or sweetcorn

Salad dressing
1 tsp sesame oil or olive oil
1 tbsp balsamic vinegar

1 tbsp lemon juice
1 tsp honey
1 tsp soya sauce
salt and freshly ground black pepper

Preparation time: 10–15 minutes.
Equipment: 1 bowl and 1 small bowl.
Storage: Fridge for 24 hours.
Servings: 2–3.

- Peel and coarsely grate the carrots, finely slice the spring onions and dice the tomatoes and avocado.
- Toss these together in the bowl with the tofu, spinach and soya beans.
- Mix the salad dressing in a small bowl, then pour over the salad.

Tofu and broccoli stir-fry

You can use baked tofu in this recipe (p160) or buy marinated tofu for ease. This goes well with noodles or brown rice.

250g baked tofu or 1 pack marinated tofu
1 carrot
100g broccoli
2 tsp rapeseed oil
3–4 mushrooms
4 spring onions
2 cloves garlic
2 tsp grated fresh root ginger
2 tsp cornflour
2 tsp reduced salt soya sauce
2 tsp honey
2 tbsp cold water

Preparation time: 15 minutes.
Equipment: 1 frying pan or wok with a lid.
Storage: Fridge for 24 hours.
Servings: 2.

- Peel and chop the carrot into matchstick-sized batons, chop the broccoli into thin bite-sized pieces and slice the mushrooms and spring onions.

- In a small bowl, mix together the cornflour, soya sauce, honey and cold water.
- Heat the oil in the pan and cook the broccoli and carrot for about 5 minutes, until softened but not quite cooked. Add a little water and put the lid on if the broccoli starts sticking to the bottom of the pan.
- Add the mushrooms, spring onions, crushed garlic and grated ginger to the pan and cook for 2 minutes.
- Add the tofu and the soya sauce mixture and cook for 2 minutes more, until everything is cooked through and the sauce has thickened.

Red lentil and vegetable stew

This is mildly spiced and Moroccan inspired with a thick, rich sauce. It goes well with rice or couscous and a spoonful of natural yogurt on top. It's a very easy, throw-it-all-in dish and you can substitute the vegetables suggested with just about anything you have in the fridge.

1 onion
1 tbsp olive oil
2 cloves garlic
1 courgette
1 red pepper
4 mushrooms
1 tsp paprika
2 tsp ground cumin
2 tsp ground coriander
1 tsp cinnamon
150g dried red lentils
1 x 400g tin chopped tomatoes
500ml stock
salt and freshly ground black pepper (optional)

Preparation time: 20 minutes plus 20 minutes cooking.
Equipment: 1 deep-sided frying pan or casserole dish with a lid.
Storage: Fridge for 24 hours or freeze.
Servings: 4.

- Peel and dice the onion.
- Cut the courgette into quarters lengthways, then slice thinly. Remove the stem and seeds from the pepper and dice. Cut the mushrooms into chunks.

- Heat the oil in the frying pan and sauté the onion and crushed garlic for 2–3 minutes over a medium heat.
- Add the courgette, peppers and mushrooms to the pan and stir, then put the lid on and leave to sweat for 5 minutes.
- Stir in the paprika, cumin, coriander and cinnamon, followed by the lentils, tomatoes and stock.
- Bring to the boil, then simmer with the lid on for about 20 minutes, until the vegetables are tender.
- Taste and add salt and pepper if you would like to.

> 66 *This was very easy to prepare and satisfying – just what was needed after a hectic day looking after two young children. We had it with couscous and a dollop of Greek yogurt and really enjoyed it.* 99
> **Rebecca, mum to Elodie, 5 months (and to Isabella, 2 years)**

Sardine pâté with lemon and parsley

A no-cook pâté that takes only 5 minutes to prepare. Ideal for busy days when you want a quick sandwich or something on toast.

1 x 120g tin sardines, preferably in olive oil
2 heaped tbsp reduced fat cream cheese (e.g. Philadelphia)
1 tsp capers
1–2 tsp lemon juice
zest of ½ a lemon
2 tbsp chopped fresh parsley
salt and pepper

Preparation time: 5 minutes.
Equipment: 1 bowl.
Storage: Fridge for 24 hours.
Servings: 2.

- Drain the sardines and mash with a fork. Remove the large bones if you prefer or just mash them in for extra calcium.
- Add the other ingredients and mash everything together thoroughly.

Fish are friends

If you don't get the reference to Disney classic *Finding Nemo*, you probably will one day soon. Fish, like friends, are particularly important to your mood and general sense of well-being when you've just had a baby. Research has shown that having a good intake of long-chain omega 3s can help improve mood and reduce the risks of post-natal depression. Including oily fish in your diet also means your breast milk will have higher levels of the long-chain omega 3 fatty acids – the healthy fats that are important for your baby's developing brain.

Fish with spiced lentils

White fish can sometimes taste quite bland, but this simple recipe transforms it into something special. You can eat it just as it is or with rice, couscous, naan bread or chapatti.

2 fillets of white fish (e.g. cod, haddock, coley)
1 small onion
2 tsp rapeseed oil
1 rounded tsp grated fresh root ginger
½ tsp ground cumin
½ tsp ground coriander
¼ tsp ground cayenne pepper
1 x 400g tin green lentils
1 tbsp tomato puree
200ml stock

To serve
wedge of lime or lemon

Preparation time: 25 minutes.
Equipment: 1 deep-sided frying pan with a lid.
Storage: Fridge for 24 hours.
Servings: 2.

- Peel and dice the onion.
- Heat the oil in the pan and sauté the onion for 3–4 minutes. Add the ginger and spices and cook for another minute.

- Drain and rinse the lentils, then add to the pan along with the tomato puree and stock. Bring to the boil, then simmer with the lid on for 10 minutes.
- Place the fish fillets on top of the lentils, put the lid back on the pan and cook for about 5 minutes, until the fish is cooked through. The amount of time needed will depend on the thickness of your fish.

Tips

- This also goes well with Indian salad (p116) or cucumber and mint raita (p123).
- Instead of adding white fish to the lentils, you could have a piece of grilled salmon.

Fact or fiction: If you eat spicy food the flavours will pass into your breast milk

It's true that if you eat food with strong flavours such as spices or garlic, then it affects the flavour of your breast milk. But don't let this put you off, as exposing babies to different flavours is one of the advantages of breastfeeding and can help reduce the chances of fussy eating. Research with adults born in Hertfordshire in the 1930s has shown that babies who were breastfed are more likely to have healthy diets when they are pensioners. The Hertfordshire-born adults who had been breastfed generally had higher intakes of fruit, vegetables, wholemeal cereals and oily fish, and lower intakes of refined cereals, sugar and full fat dairy produce. Research in the past has shown that when babies are weaned, they're more likely to accept particular flavours that their mum has eaten while breastfeeding, but the Hertfordshire research suggests that the benefits of flavour-learning from breast milk are extremely long lasting. It also seems that exposing babies to flavour compounds from their mother's diet tends to increase their preferences for the flavours found in more natural and more healthy foods. Don't go mad, though, and start eating spicy chillies and hot curries – a sudden and dramatic change in the flavour of breast milk can put babies off feeding or cause tummy upsets. Just enjoy a wide range of flavours so that your baby will too.

Speedy prawn noodles

This is a quick version of pad thai and combines flat rice noodles with prawns, beansprouts, peanuts and lime juice. It involves very little chopping so doesn't take as long to prepare as a regular stir-fry, and it uses ingredients that can be bought in any supermarket so it's an easy midweek meal.

125g rice noodles
5 spring onions
2 tsp rapeseed oil
handful frozen soya beans or peas
200g beansprouts
2 tsp soya sauce
1 tbsp sweet chilli sauce
1 egg
150g prawns
3–4 tbsp fresh coriander
2 tbsp chopped peanuts
¼ lime

Preparation time: 15 minutes.
Equipment: 1 frying pan or wok and a pan for noodles.
Storage: Fridge for 24 hours.
Servings: 2.

- Cook the noodles according to the instructions on the packet.
- Finely slice the spring onions.
- Heat the oil in the frying pan and add the spring onions, soya beans or peas, beansprouts, soya sauce and chilli sauce. Stir-fry for 3–4 minutes on a high heat.
- Move the vegetables to the edges of the pan and crack the egg into the centre. Stir the egg for a minute or so, until it is lightly scrambled, then add the noodles and prawns to the pan and cook for a few minutes, until everything is steaming hot.
- Add the coriander and serve with chopped nuts sprinkled on top and a squeeze of lime juice.

Spaghetti with salmon and red pesto

This makes a quick and easy midweek meal that includes oily fish, tastes delicious and provides all the nutrients your growing baby needs.

150g spaghetti
2 salmon fillets or steaks
12 cherry tomatoes
2 tbsp sliced black olives
2 tbsp red pesto
2 tbsp ricotta

Preparation time: 20 minutes.
Equipment: 1 large pan and 1 baking tray.
Storage: Eat straightaway.
Servings: 2.

- Put the spaghetti in a large pan of boiling water.
- Place the salmon fillets on a baking tray covered with tin foil and grill under a medium heat for about 5 minutes on each side.
- Meanwhile, wash the cherry tomatoes and cut them in half.
- When the salmon is ready, remove the skin and discard, then gently flake the fish into large chunks.
- Drain the spaghetti and, over a low heat, stir through the salmon, tomatoes, olives, pesto and ricotta.

Tip

- You can also add frozen peas or some cooked mange tout or asparagus.

66 *Quick, yummy and very little to wash up – perfect! My 6-year-old enjoyed it and said it was the best meal I have cooked.* 99
Kerry, mum to Myrie, 13 months (and to Rose, 6 years, and David, 4 years)

How to stock up on healthy foods

Things don't always go to plan when you've got a new baby to look after. Popping to the shops can become a major operation, and even organising a sensible online delivery isn't always possible. So it's good to stock up on staples that you can throw together to create an easy but reasonably healthy meal. Good foods for the cupboard include: tins of tomatoes, chickpeas, kidney beans, tuna and sardines; packets of pasta, rice and couscous; and something to add flavour, such as mixed herbs, stock cubes, lemon juice and soya sauce. If you have some frozen vegetables, fish and maybe some minced meat in the freezer, then you'll never, or hardly ever, need to rely on the local takeaway or have toast for dinner. Ideally, your fridge will be stocked with fresh food too, including fruit and vegetables, but don't worry if you can't always manage that.

Italian chicken baked with tomatoes and olives

This is a variation of the Italian cacciatore stew, which is usually made with wine. It looks after itself in the oven, so it's ready when you are. Great with rice, baked potatoes or new potatoes, and green beans.

250g diced chicken
1 onion
2 tsp olive oil
2 cloves garlic
2 tbsp white wine vinegar
1 x 400g tin chopped tomatoes
1 tbsp tomato puree
1 tsp dried basil or 1 tbsp fresh basil
1 tsp dried parsley or 1 tbsp fresh parsley
1 bay leaf
2 tbsp pitted black olives, whole or sliced
salt and freshly ground black pepper

Preparation time: 15 minutes plus 30 minutes baking.
Equipment: 1 ovenproof pan or casserole dish with a lid.
Storage: Fridge for 24 hours.
Servings: 2.

- Preheat the oven to 180°C (160°C fan)/350°F/gas mark 4.
- Peel and finely dice the onion.
- Heat the oil in the pan and fry the chicken for a few minutes to brown the outside, then remove it from the pan.
- Add the onion and crushed garlic to the pan and cook for about 5 minutes, until soft.
- Add the vinegar to deglaze the pan and stir in any brown bits from the bottom. Add the tomatoes, tomato puree, basil, parsley, bay leaf and olives. Stir, then return the chicken to the pan. Bring to the boil, then place in the oven for 30 minutes.
- Add some black pepper and a little salt if needed.

Tip

- You can also add extra vegetables, such as mushrooms or peppers, and other herbs – rosemary also works well.

66 *This was really quick and easy to prepare and everyone enjoyed it. I used three chicken breasts and that did us all, which was really good, as often I will be cooking three different meals in the evening. I pureed Miranda's and mixed it with rice – again, which we all had.* 99

Lara, mum to Miranda, 10 months (and to Vanessa, 3 years)

Sunday roast lamb all-in-one

Roast lamb steaks and all the trimmings, including real gravy, with only 20 minutes' preparation, 30 minutes in the oven and hardly any washing up. Cooking a roast couldn't be easier.

2 lamb steaks, trimmed of fat
2 tsp rapeseed oil
2 carrots
2 parsnips
350g new potatoes
1 tsp chopped fresh rosemary or ½ tsp dried rosemary
250ml stock
1 tsp cornflour mixed with 1 tbsp cold water
1 tbsp red wine vinegar
150g peas
2 mint leaves

Preparation time: 20 minutes plus 30 minutes roasting.
Equipment: 1 roasting tin and 1 bowl.
Storage: Fridge for 24 hours.
Servings: 2.

- Preheat the oven to 220°C (200°C fan)/425°F/gas mark 7.
- Peel the carrots and parsnips and chop into 2cm thick chunks. The fat ends of the vegetables may also need to be cut in half lengthways.
- Slice the potatoes into 1cm thick slices.
- Place 1 teaspoon of oil in the roasting tin and place it on the cooker over a medium heat. Cook the lamb steaks for 2 minutes on each side to brown, then set them aside on a plate.
- Put the other teaspoon of oil into the roasting tin, then put in the chopped carrots and parsnips and sliced potatoes and toss to coat them in the

oil. Spread everything out into a single layer and place in the oven for 10 minutes.

- Give the vegetables a stir, then place the lamb steaks on top and the chopped rosemary. Return to the oven for 20 minutes, until the lamb is cooked through and the vegetables are tender.
- Prepare the stock and the cornflour mixture. Place the peas in a microwaveable bowl with the torn mint leaves and a tablespoon of water, but don't cook them yet.
- Turn the oven off, then move everything from the roasting tin into a serving dish and place in the oven to keep warm while you make the gravy.
- Heat the roasting tin on top of the cooker over a medium heat and add the stock and vinegar. Using a wooden spoon, stir the gently bubbling liquid and scrape the bottom of the tin for 2–3 minutes. Add the cornflour mixture and stir for another minute to thicken the gravy, then turn off the heat.
- Cook the peas in the microwave for 2–3 minutes, until hot.
- Pour the gravy into a jug and get the roast lamb, potatoes and vegetables out of the oven.

Tip

- If you're cooking for more people, you'll need to use another roasting tin or baking tray so that the ingredients can lie in a single layer, otherwise you'll need to increase the cooking time by about 20 minutes.

> 66 *This was a very tasty meal that we all enjoyed. We doubled up the ingredients so there was enough for us all.* 99
> **Kerry, mum to Myrie, 13 months (and to Rose, 6 years, and David, 4 years)**

Fact or fiction: Beer is good for breastfeeding

It's fine to have one beer or a glass of wine but it's a myth that it helps with breastfeeding. It used to be said that Guinness was good because it contains lots of iron (which it doesn't, by the way) or that beer in general improved milk supply. However, research has shown that when women have even one alcoholic drink, their baby has to work harder to get some milk and tends to drink less. This is because alcohol affects the let-down reflex in the breast that usually makes it easier for the baby to feed.

Stir-fried pork with green peppers

Stir-fried pork and green peppers with soya sauce, ginger and honey. An ideal midweek supper with rice or noodles.

250g pork tenderloin or loin (or use diced stir-fry pork or leftover roast pork)
2 tsp cornflour
1 tbsp reduced salt soya sauce
1 tbsp honey
2 tbsp water
2 tsp rapeseed oil
1 green pepper
150g cabbage (green, savoy or sweetheart)
1 tbsp grated fresh root ginger
2 cloves garlic

Preparation time: 15 minutes.
Equipment: 1 frying pan.
Storage: Fridge for 24 hours or freeze.
Servings: 2.

- Cut the pork into bite-sized cubes or strips.
- In a small bowl, mix together the cornflour, soya sauce, honey and water.
- Remove the stalk and seeds from the pepper and slice thinly. Shred the cabbage and prepare the grated ginger and crushed garlic. It's good to have everything ready so that you can add them when needed and don't overcook the pork.
- Heat the oil in the frying pan over a high heat. Fry the pork for 2 minutes, until browned all over.
- Add the pepper, cabbage, garlic and ginger and cook for a further 3–4 minutes, until the vegetables are cooked.
- Give the cornflour mixture a stir, then pour it into the pan, turn the heat down and stir for a minute to thicken.

> 66 *I loved this stir-fry recipe. Really tasty and easy to follow. I tried it with chicken and beef too and they worked just as well and were also delicious.* 99
> **Sarah, mum to Georgia, 3 months**

Meatloaf

This is packed with flavour but economical and very easy to make. Serve with baked potatoes, carrots and broccoli or green beans. You can also make it ahead of time while your baby naps and keep it in the fridge ready to pop in the oven later on.

2 tsp olive oil or rapeseed oil, plus extra for greasing
1 onion
2 cloves garlic
1 carrot
2 mushrooms
400g lean minced beef
50g fresh breadcrumbs (wholemeal or white)
2 tbsp tomato puree
1 egg
20g Parmesan cheese or similar hard cheese
2 tsp Worcestershire sauce
1 tsp mixed herbs
salt and pepper

Preparation time: 20 minutes plus 1 hour baking.
Equipment: 1 frying pan, 1 mixing bowl and a 2lb loaf tin (about 22cm x 11cm internally).
Storage: Fridge for 24 hours or freeze.
Servings: 4.

- Preheat the oven to 200°C (180°C fan)/400°F/gas mark 6.
- Grease a loaf tin and line with greaseproof paper.
- Peel and dice the onion.
- Heat the oil in the frying pan and sauté the onion with the crushed garlic for 5 minutes.
- Meanwhile, peel and finely dice the carrot and dice the mushrooms. Add to the onion and cook for 5 more minutes.
- Place the minced beef, breadcrumbs, tomato puree, egg, grated cheese, Worcestershire sauce, herbs and some salt and pepper in a mixing bowl.
- Add the cooked vegetables to the bowl, then combine all the ingredients using one hand.
- Transfer the mixture to the loaf tin and press it down. Place in the oven for 1 hour, until nicely browned on top and completely cooked through. Or,

once it's in the tin, you can cover it with cling film and put it in the fridge to cook later.

Why you should eat plenty of zinc

Zinc is an essential part of many of our hormones. It is needed for the formation of healthy new cells and for the proper functioning of the immune system. During pregnancy, you needed 7mg of zinc per day, the same amount recommended for all women. However, during breastfeeding this increases to 13mg a day. This is quite a substantial increase, so it's important to ensure that you eat plenty of zinc-rich foods such as beef and other meat, milk, cheese and yogurt. Zinc is also found in cereal products, but if you eat refined products you'll get much less than you would from wholegrain foods. Two slices of wholemeal bread, for example, will provide you with 1.3mg of zinc, whereas the same amount of white bread contains only 0.5mg. Swapping regular pasta for brown and breakfast cereals such as cornflakes for branflakes will also provide you with extra zinc, as well as increasing your intake of fibre and other minerals.

Desserts and snacks

Why you should eat bananas

Bananas are the most popular fruit in the UK and it's easy to see why: they're sweet, conveniently packaged in their own skin and healthy. Bananas are rich in potassium, which helps counteract the effects of sodium and maintain a healthy blood pressure. They also contain fructooligosaccharide, a form of carbohydrate that isn't digested in the normal way but instead acts as a prebiotic and provides food for the friendly bacteria in the gut. This in turn can improve immunity, bone health and the overall balance of bacteria in the digestive tract. So reach for a banana instead of a biscuit to give you and your baby a real health boost.

Crunchy fruit pot

Pineapple, mango, kiwi or any of your favourite fruits with yogurt and a crunchy coconut topping.

¼ fresh pineapple
½ ripe mango
1 kiwi
2 tbsp porridge oats
2 tbsp desiccated coconut
2 tsp dark muscovado sugar
2 tbsp raisins
200g low fat natural yogurt or reduced fat Greek yogurt

Preparation time: 15 minutes.
Equipment: 1 small frying pan.
Storage: Eat straightaway.
Servings: 2.

- Peel and dice the fruit into 1cm pieces and divide between two dessert bowls.
- In a frying pan, heat the porridge oats and coconut for 2–3 minutes stirring occasionally, until just starting to brown, then remove from the heat.
- Add the sugar and raisins to the pan and stir.
- Spoon the yogurt over the fruit, then sprinkle the coconut topping over the top.

Tip

- You can use any fruit in this dish – fresh banana with a squeeze of lime juice works well.

Eton mess

A sweet and creamy dessert that makes a lovely treat without too many calories and more than a portion of fruit each.

150g fat-free Greek yogurt
4 tbsp half-fat crème fraîche
200g strawberries
2 meringue nests

Preparation time: 10 minutes.
Equipment: 1 bowl.
Storage: Fridge for 24 hours.
Servings: 2.

- Mix together the Greek yogurt and crème fraîche.
- Slice the strawberries and stir into the mixture.
- Break the meringue nests into small pieces. Just before serving, stir gently into the yogurt mixture. You can make the strawberry mixture and leave it in the fridge but, once mixed in, the meringues lose their crunch after a while.

Tip

- Instead of using half fat crème fraîche, which is about 15% fat, you could use low fat crème fraîche, which is just 3% fat. If you do this, you might want to use 'low fat' Greek yogurt instead of 'fat free' Greek yogurt. Having some fat in the mixture helps provide a creamy texture, but by choosing reduced fat products you won't be overloading with calories and saturated fat.

Quick and easy fruit cake

This takes only 15 minutes to prepare, and even if you've never baked before you can't go wrong. Ideal with an afternoon cup of tea when energy levels are flagging and healthier than shop-bought alternatives, as it contains a mixture of wholemeal and white flour and is made with rapeseed oil instead of butter or margarine.

125g wholemeal flour
125g plain flour
4 tsp baking powder
100g soft brown sugar
1 tsp ground mixed spice
250g mixed dried fruit
2 eggs
125ml rapeseed oil
150ml milk
1 tsp demerara sugar

Preparation time: 15 minutes plus 50 minutes baking.
Equipment: 1 mixing bowl and a 2lb loaf tin or round cake tin (20cm–25cm diameter).
Storage: Airtight container for 2–3 days or freeze.
Servings: 1 large cake.

- Preheat the oven to 180°C (160°C fan)/350°F/gas mark 4. Grease the loaf or cake tin and line the bottom with greaseproof paper.
- In the mixing bowl, combine the flours, baking powder, soft brown sugar, mixed spice and dried fruit.
- Push the ingredients to the sides of the bowl to make a well in the centre.
- Crack the eggs into the centre of the bowl and pour in the oil and milk.
- Lightly beat the wet ingredients using a fork. Then, using a spoon, bring in the dry ingredients and mix well to combine everything.
- Transfer the mixture to the prepared tin, smooth it over, and sprinkle with the spoonful of demerara sugar.
- Bake for about 50 minutes, until a skewer inserted in the centre comes out dry.
- Leave to cool in the tin for 5–10 minutes before taking it out and leaving on a cooling rack.

Tips

- If the top browns too much before the centre is cooked, loosely place a piece of foil over the top.
- You can easily adapt this basic recipe and replace the mixed dried fruit with sultanas, apricots, dates or even some chopped nuts.
- You can also add 1–2 tsp ground ginger to the recipe.

Apricot and almond cake

This is a delicious and beautifully moist cake. The recipe is wheat free, as oats and ground almonds are used instead of regular wheat flour. The almonds also supply extra calcium for strong bones and vitamin E for healthy skin, while the apricots will help boost your iron intake.

125g oats
150ml orange juice
150g dried apricots
3 eggs
50ml rapeseed oil plus extra for greasing
125g ground almonds
100g soft brown sugar
2 tsp baking powder
1 tsp ground mixed spice

Preparation time: 20 minutes plus 25–30 minutes baking.
Equipment: 1 mixing bowl and 1 loose-based cake tin (23cm diameter).
Storage: Airtight container for a few days or freeze.
Servings: 10.

- Put the oats into the mixing bowl, pour the orange juice over them and leave to soak.
- Preheat the oven to 180°C (160°C fan)/350°F/gas mark 4. Grease the cake tin and line the bottom with greaseproof paper.
- Cut the dried apricots by making a mound on a chopping board and roughly chopping them into pea-sized pieces.
- Place the oil in a measuring jug. Add the eggs and beat.
- Add the ground almonds, sugar, baking powder and mixed spice to the oats, then stir.
- Add the egg and oil mixture and stir again so that all the ingredients are well mixed.
- Pour the mixture into the prepared tin and bake for about 25–30 minutes, until a skewer inserted in the centre comes out dry.
- Leave to cool for 5 minutes before removing from the tin and peeling off the greaseproof paper, then leave on a cooling rack until completely cool.

Fact or fiction: You can eat what you like when you're breastfeeding because you need the extra calories

Breastfeeding inevitably uses up calories, but this doesn't mean you can snack on chocolate and biscuits all day without putting on weight. Some women find they lose weight naturally and gradually while they're breastfeeding, but others feel more hungry than usual and find it difficult to shed the post-pregnancy pounds. If you need to lose weight, don't skip meals or restrict your calorie intake too much as this can reduce your milk supply. However, research has shown that losing about 1–2 pounds a week is fine while breastfeeding. If you find you're losing weight too quickly or if you're a healthy weight and feel hungry between meals, try not to turn to sugary snacks. It's fine to have them sometimes, but healthy snacks such as a bowl of cereal or some wholemeal toast with houmous or cream cheese are much more nutritious. If you want something sweeter, then malt loaf, hot cross buns and fig rolls are good choices.

Cranberry and pumpkin seed squares

These are like cereal bars but without all the added sugar that you find in most of those you can buy.

2 ripe bananas
200g porridge oats
50g dried cranberries
50g pumpkin seeds
100ml rapeseed oil
3 tbsp honey

Preparation time: 10 minutes plus 20 minutes cooking.
Equipment: 1 baking tray (approximately 20cm x 30cm x 2cm) and 1 mixing bowl.
Storage: Airtight container for 3–4 days or freeze.
Servings: 24 squares.

- Preheat the oven to 180°C (160°C fan)/350°F/gas mark 4.
- Cover the baking tray with a piece of greaseproof paper. This doesn't need to be cut to size but can overhang the edges.
- Slice the bananas into the mixing bowl, then mash with a potato masher or fork.
- Stir in the oats, pumpkin seeds, cranberries, honey and oil.
- Spoon the mixture into the prepared tin and press down well with the back of your spoon to make an even layer.
- Bake for 20 minutes, until golden brown.
- Take it out of the oven and mark into 24 squares.
- Leave until completely cool, then slice through and put the squares into an airtight container.

Tip

- You can make these with other seeds or nuts instead of pumpkin seeds and try crystallised ginger or other dried fruit such as raisins or apricots.

Cheddar scones

These are great warm from the oven with a bowl of soup, or have them as a snack to boost your calcium intake.

> 100g wholemeal flour
> 100g plain flour, plus extra for dusting
> 25g oats
> 1 tbsp baking powder
> 100g reduced fat Cheddar cheese
> 1 tsp Dijon mustard
> 50ml rapeseed oil, plus extra for greasing
> 150ml milk

Preparation time: 10 minutes plus 10–15 minutes baking.
Equipment: 1 baking tray and 1 mixing bowl.
Storage: Airtight container for a few days or freeze.
Servings: 12 scones.

- Preheat the oven to 220°C (200°C fan)/425°F/gas mark 7. Lightly grease a baking tray.
- In a mixing bowl, place the flour, oats and baking power.
- Grate the cheese into the bowl but save about one tablespoonful for later.
- Stir the mixture and make a well in the centre, then add the mustard, oil and milk.
- Stir with a spoon to form a dough, then, using your hands, bring the dough together to form a ball.
- Place on a floured work surface and roll to a thickness of about 2cm.
- Cut into circles 5cm across using a biscuit cutter.
- Place the scones on the baking tray and bake for 10–15 minutes.

Drinks

Chocolate thick shake

This is thick and creamy but much healthier than the average shake. You can't taste the avocado but it provides creaminess and healthy monounsaturated fats.

> 225ml milk
> 2 tsp cocoa powder
> 1 tbsp maple syrup
> ½ small/medium avocado

Preparation time: 5 minutes.
Pans: 1 blender.
Storage: Fridge for 24 hours.
Servings: 1.

- Place everything in the blender and blend until smooth.

Tip

- If you don't have any maple syrup, use honey or caster sugar instead.

Breastfeeding meal planner

This meal planner shows what a healthy diet for breastfeeding looks like. Your exact nutrient requirements will depend on how much milk your baby is having (p149). As well as plenty of fruit, vegetables and starchy carbohydrate-rich foods, it includes healthy snacks to supply the extra nutrients your body needs to produce milk.

This meal plan meets the requirements for protein, potassium, calcium, magnesium, phosphorus, iron, copper, zinc, chloride, selenium, iodine, thiamin, riboflavin, niacin and vitamins A, B6, B12, C and E.

To meet all the nutrient requirements for breastfeeding, you should also take a supplement containing 10µg vitamin D (see p150) and have plenty of water and other fluids to drink.

Day 1

Breakfast: Fruit salad and yoghurt, 2 slices of toast and almond butter
Lunch: Corn chowder (p156), granary bread, Cheddar, a pear
Dinner: Italian chicken baked with tomatoes and olives (p169), baked potato, strawberries and dairy ice cream
Snacks: Fruit bun, a banana, wholemeal pitta with houmous

Day 2

Breakfast: Large bowl of muesli and milk, a crumpet with honey
Lunch: Sardine pâté with lemon and parsley (p164) on wholemeal toast, tomato, cucumber, a pot of low fat yogurt

Dinner: Vegetarian sausages, new potatoes, broccoli, carrots and ketchup, crunchy fruit pot (p174)
Snacks: Grapes, 2 Weetabix with milk, 2 slices of malt loaf

Day 3

Breakfast: Tomato poached eggs (p153), wholemeal toast
Lunch: 2 chicken drumsticks, Mediterranean couscous salad (p113), houmous, carrot sticks
Dinner: Spaghetti with salmon and red pesto (p167), mixed salad, fruit salad and yogurt
Snacks: 2 crumpets with fruit spread, a handful of Brazil nuts

Day 4

Breakfast: Large bowl of fruit and fibre cereal with milk, strawberry and yogurt smoothie (p154)
Lunch: Spanish omelette, granary bread, mixed salad
Dinner: Red lentil and vegetable stew (p163), rice and low fat yogurt, chocolate cake and ice cream
Snacks: Large bowl of muesli, quick and easy fruit cake (p176), an apple

Day 5

Breakfast: Large bowl of branflakes with yogurt and raspberries
Lunch: Large baked potato with baked beans and cheese, an orange
Dinner: Sunday roast lamb all-in-one (p170), pear and ginger breakfast crumble (p18) and custard
Snacks: 2 slices of wholemeal toast and yeast extract, quick and easy fruit cake (p176)

Day 6

Breakfast: Muesli, granary toast with honey
Lunch: Baked tofu salad (p161), mixed salad
Dinner: Fish with spiced lentils (p165), couscous, Indian salad (p116), fruit salad and frozen yoghurt
Snacks: Chocolate thick shake (p180), wholemeal pitta and houmous, fig roll biscuits

Day 7

Breakfast: Carrot cake porridge (p63)
Lunch: Ham and salad wholemeal sandwich, crunchy fruit pot (p174)
Dinner: Corn on the cob, cheese and tomato pizza, salad
Snacks: Cheddar scones (p179), grapes, yogurt

Alphabetical list of recipes

Alphabetical list of recipes

This is Pregnancy, but

FOR MEN

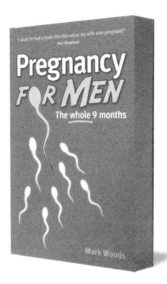

A comprehensive and utterly honest guide designed
to help men navigate the choppy waters of pregnancy.
Taking the whole thing a month at a time and using the
experiences of scores of first time Dads, this is a frank,
factual and funny journey charting what men need to
know when their partners are pregnant.

Follow us on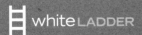

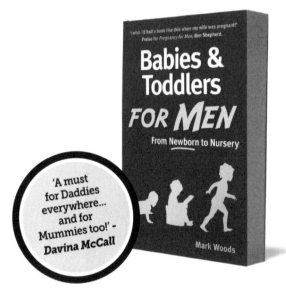

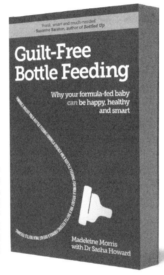
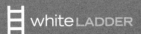

All you need to know about spoon feeding and baby-led weaning – get the best of both worlds

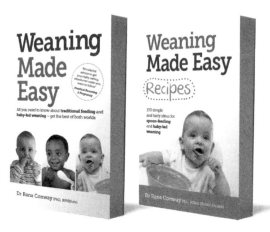

Weaning Made Easy uses the best of each method, to bring you the most practical and useful weaning advice available. From what foods to try (and avoid) in the first six months to moving your baby onto family meals, Rana Conway covers it all.

Weaning Made Easy Recipes has 150 tasty recipes to suit all babies, toddlers and approaches. Whether you find that your baby loves being spoon-fed, only wants to feed themselves, or you want to try a mixture of both, *Weaning Made Easy Recipes* has a range of healthy meals to make mealtimes enjoyable for everyone.

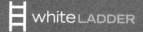